Praise for

Till We Eat Again

"From resolution to reunion, through calorie deprivation and tortuous perspiration, Judy takes us on a very funny aerobic ride in her quest for inner esteem and outer svelte."

W. Bruce Cameron, nationally syndicated columnist and author of *8 Simple Rules for Dating My Teenage Daughter*

"Judy Gruen has done it again! In her signature comic fashion, she captures the true essence of the whole dieting game—and how crazy we are for continually falling for all the empty promises and quick fixes. Through Judy's journey to svelthood, she discovers what she really knew all along—that true wellness goes way beyond some number on a weight chart and comes from moderation in all things, including chocolate; that a stronger body comes from a little hard work, not a pill or an electronic belt; and that there is humor in almost every situation, even if it means laughing at yourself. Before you fall for the next big weight loss scheme, gadget, or pill, read this! It'll be the last 'diet' book you'll ever need."

Carrie Myers Smith, columnist for *Energy* magazine, president of *WomenInWellness.com*

"Judy Gruen is hilarious! In *Till We Eat Again* we follow Judy through her trials (and errors) of losing weight. When the scales refuse to budge and she runs for comfort to a bag of chocolates, we really feel her pain! What woman can't relate to this?"

Debbie Farmer, syndicated columnist, author of *Life in the Fast Food Lane*

"If you can imagine a humor book as page turner, then you can imagine *Till We Eat Again*. . .Judy has the Dave Barry touch—her sentences take unexpected turns that have you clutching your sides with laughter while keeping your eyes glued to the pages."

Kathy Fitzgerald Sherman author of *A Housekeeper Is Cheaper Than a Divorce*

Till We Eat Again

confessions of a diet dropout

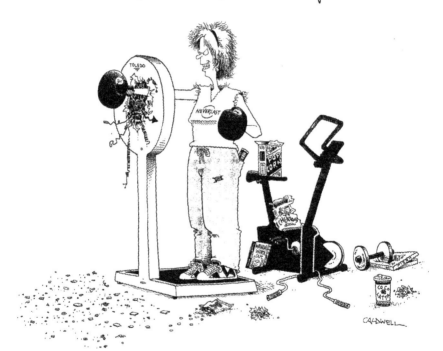

Till We Eat Again

confessions of a diet dropout

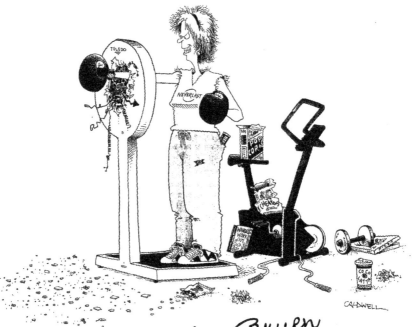

Judy Gruen

CHAMPION PRESS LTD.

Milwaukee, Wisconsin

ALSO BY JUDY GRUEN

CARPOOL TUNNEL SYNDROME:
MOTHERHOOD AS SHUTTLE DIPLOMACY

OFF MY NOODLE
FREE SEMI-MONTHLY HUMOR COLUMN
to subscribe visit www.judygruen.com

CHAMPION PRESS, LTD.
MILWAUKEE, WISCONSIN

For more information contact: Champion Press, Ltd., 4308 Blueberry Road, Fredonia, WI 53021, www.championpress.com

LCCN 2002111688
ISBN 1-891400-92-4
Manufactured in the United States of America 10 9 8 7 6 5 4 3
Book Cover Illustration by Johnny Caldwell
Book Cover and Book Design by Pilot Publishing
Author Photograph by Daryl Tempkin
Inside Illustrations by Johnny Caldwell

For Jeff—
My only one, now and forever.

ACKNOWLEDGMENTS

Special thanks to Brook Noel of Champion Press for her enthusiasm and hard work in helping this book become a reality. My gratitude also to the other good folks at Champion Press, including Kim Meiloch, Mary Ann Koopmann, Joan Egan, and Michael Gulan, Wendy Feiereisen and Anne Peiffer for their very important work, done cheerfully and unflaggingly, in helping to bring new books to life and promoting them once they're here.

Leanne Ely, Denise Koek, Brook Noel, Jeff Gruen and Noah Gruen all made valuable editorial suggestions and seemed to laugh at the right places. Thank you.

A big "Hoo-Yah!" to Jay Kerwin ("The Major"), who gave me a new respect for the military and who helped me discover that I really could do toes-down push-ups. And finally, this book would not have been possible without the other innumerable exercise instructors, nutrition experts, colonic irrigators, hypnotherapists, yoga teachers and other people who gave me unbelievably funny material without even trying. Keep up the good work. I may do a sequel.

Contents

3   / PREFACE... Curl Up and Diet

5   / NOVEMBER ... Let Me Eat Cake!

18 / DECEMBER ... Waist Not, Want Not

40 / JANUARY ... Bound for Glory

57 / FEBRUARY ... Mission: Improbable

83 / MARCH ... Belly Dancing, Boxing and the Bread of Affliction

104 / APRIL... Guru Hari and the Forty Thieves

139 / MAY ... Sweat Gets in My Eyes, But I Also Get New Clothes

159 / JUNE ... Stand and Deliver

180 / NOVEMBER ... Against All Odds

Preface

Curl Up and Diet
By Ogden Nash

Some ladies smoke too much and some ladies drink too
 much and some ladies pray too much,
But all ladies think that they weigh too much.
They may be as slender as a sylph or a dryad,
But just let them get on the scales and they embark on a doleful jer-
emiad;
No matter how low the figure on the needle happens to touch,
They always claim it is at least five pounds too much;
To the world she may appear slinky and feline,
But she inspects herself in the mirror and cries, Oh, I look like a sea lion;
Yes, she tells you she is growing into the shape of a sea cow or manatee,
And if you say No, my dear, she says you are just lying
 to make her feel better,
And if you say Yes, my dear you injure her vanity.
Once upon a time there was a girl more beautiful and
 witty and charming than tongue could tell,
And she is now a dangerous raving maniac in a padded cell,
And the first indication her relatives had that
 she was mentally overwrought was one day when she said I weigh a
hundred
 and twenty-seven, which is exactly what I ought.
Oh, often I am haunted
By the thought that somebody might discover
A diet that would let ladies reduce just as much as they wanted,
Because I wonder if there is a woman in the world
Strong-minded enough to shed ten pounds or twenty,
And say There now, that's plenty;
And I fear me one ten-pound loss would only arouse the
 craving for another

So it wouldn't do any good for ladies to get their ambition
and look like somebody's fourteen-year-old brother,
Because, having accomplished this with ease,
They would next want to look like somebody's fourteen-
year-old brother in the final stages of some obscure
disease,
And the more success you have the more you want to
get of it
So then their goal would be to look like somebody's
fourteen-year-old brother's ghost, or rather not the
ghost itself, which is fairly solid, but a silhouette
of it,
So I think it is very nice for ladies to be lithe and lissome,
But not so much that you cut yourself if you happen
to embrace or kissome.

NOVEMBER

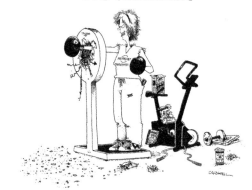

Let Me Eat Cake!

November 5

I am hugely relieved to report that my friend Ingrid has just left the house after a weeklong visit, taking her soy milk and ankle weights with her. Having Ingrid in the house for a week was like running a bed and breakfast for low-fat guru Covert Bailey. Since I had last seen her two years ago, Ingrid has gotten religion and now bows to the gods of organic kale and Kundulani yoga. Unfortunately, she now also resembles those missionaries who come to the door early Saturday mornings, ready to witness to you.

Even before she unpacked, Ingrid had scanned the contents of my pantry, her lips curling in disapproval. Sighing, she asked for directions to the nearest organic market, and dashed off to Seven Grain Heaven. She breezed back an hour later, invigorated by the aroma of sizzling gluten steaks in the store's take-out section. Ingrid's taut and toned arms were laden with two bags full of exotic health food, including chicken-less chicken, egg-less eggs, rainforest vegan cookies made with real barley malt, and bread that was surprisingly heavy considering that it had no flour, yeast, salt, sugar, oil, or any other ingredients. We put away this bounty of nutrient-charged provisions on a shelf I had "cleared" of two of our family's two main food groups: potato chips and snack cookies, whose most vital ingredients were refined white sugar and BHT.

On the second morning of her visit Ingrid strode purposefully into the kitchen during breakfast, while the kids were pouring an avalanche of Sugar-Cocoa-Yum cereal into bowls. Surveying this scene, Ingrid offered to share her own breakfast of steel-cut oats with me. I declined, worried the cereal might chip the enamel off my teeth.

As I sat down with my own bowl of whole-grain cereal (sprinkled, I admit, with some cookie crumbs that would otherwise have gone to waste), Ingrid warned, "That lump of refined carbohydrates may make you *think* you're full, but your body will still be starving for nutrients." She then confidently stirred her steel-cut oats to their bland conclusion. I had known Ingrid since college, and was seized with jealousy that she now wore jeans two sizes smaller than she had worn in those good old days, when our idea of an adventure was hunting through the frozen foods section of the supermarket, plotting our next rendezvous with Sara Lee, Ben & Jerry, and other comrades. Back in college, Ingrid used to rail that fitness was "a patriarchal social construct." Why had she turned on me?

As she spoke, I took a large swig of my coffee and defiantly spooned up another mouthful of my vitamin-challenged cereal, suddenly craving a big hunk of chocolate chunk brownie. With our visit less than twenty-four hours old, Ingrid was already getting on my nerves. She had lost the fifteen pounds that I hadn't, and fairly burst with vitality. Meanwhile, I pondered my day's schedule, trying to see when I could possibly sneak in a nap. I stole a glance at Ingrid as she poured a thick steaming gruel into her bowl, and wondered if she would let me use the leftovers to spackle the hallway.

Unfortunately, things got worse. At six a.m. on day three of her visit, I heard a knock at the door. I ambled down the hall with my eyes barely peeled open, only to find Ingrid unbuckling her inline skates on the porch. She was glistening from a six-mile blading excursion through the neighborhood.

"So glad I got an early start!," she chirped. "Did you know rollerblading burns 400 calories an hour?"

I waved her in and started up the coffee, sick in the knowledge that at this ungodly hour I was already 400 calories behind schedule. I comforted myself that if nothing else, at least Ingrid and I still shared a love of fresh-brewed coffee. Over her steaming cup of joe and mound of steel cut oats, she told me about a great recipe for a seven-layer carob cake, but I tuned out after hearing the first three layers were flaxseed, prune puree and lecithin. I wondered what kind of twisted mind would think up something like this. While images of glazed donuts danced in my head, I began to worry, "Could this friendship be saved?"

November 6

The question gnawed at me until I snuck out later that day wearing dark shades for a midday burger and fries. Thanks to Ingrid, I had been reduced to eating incognito. Blast! Why didn't I have her sense of discipline? Her commitment to exercise? Her respect for arugula?

That afternoon, before I had even fully digested my lunch, Ingrid asked, "Say, Judy, have you heard about the Coop reunion this summer? Can you believe it will have been twenty years since you and I moved out and graduated from the U?" The Coop was the small, independent cooperative dorm where we both lived during college. The building housed about thirty students and a few recent graduates who continued to hang around, stalling for time before figuring out whether to capitulate and join the family business selling fabric linings, or to extort more money from their folks for law school.

Since we allowed more students to live there than was legal, life in the Coop fostered a certain ill-advised intimacy among many housemates, some of whom had nothing more in common than that both were waiting to use the washing machine at the same time. In these hothouse circumstances, relationships often blossomed while laundry was loaded into the machine but had flailed into oblivion by the last spin cycle. Ah, the recklessness of youth!

"Twenty years! Hard to believe it's been that long!" I said. "Do you have any idea how many people might show?" I was curious. It would be fun to see a lot of Coop pals – friends like Lana, a real live wire who not only aced all her finals without seeming to study, but also worked weekends as a cook in one of the restaurants near the U. But I especially wondered about the two housemates who had broken my heart in rapid succession, and whom I had lost track of completely. First was Gary, with his drop-dead gorgeous blue eyes and mischievous grin, who never realized that I was in love with him. I waited in vain for him to drop that mousy, humorless, Save-the-Whales girlfriend of his, but by the time they split up, we had all graduated and gone our separate ways.

And then of course there was that cad, Hartley, who eventually pushed me into the arms of a therapist after he discarded me like so much used notebook paper. If ever a name should have warned me off, it should have been a guy named Hartley! But at the beginning of my senior year when Hartley moved into the house, I was a goner at first glance. Hartley seemed to possess the most important qualities that any young woman would want in a young man, namely, a rakishly handsome face and blonde hair. But to top it off, Hartley's impromptu recitals of Shakespearian sonnets and scenes from *As You Like It* rendered me incapable of focusing on anything other than him. Hartley had wit, brains, and vanity galore, but at the time I thought his vanity was a small price to pay for a guy who would look meaningfully into my eyes as if I were the only girl in the world and declare, "Shall I compare thee to a summer's day? Thou art more lovely and more temperate. . ." Besides, what else did I expect from a theater arts major?

In my standard college uniform of appallingly unflattering denim overalls that covered a chunky physique, it may have been unrealistic to expect a guy like Hartley to fall for me. So it may have been just coincidence that we dated for the six months during which Hartley rehearsed a play that he had written and directed, and I had offered to become his backstage gofer. I ran to get coffee whenever the actors wanted some, helped to paint stage scenery, made copies of new script pages, anything that would make Hartley's life easier. The play was a smashing success. My grades that semester simply smashed.

As far as I was concerned, this devotion on my part made Hartley and me as good as married. But Hartley had other ideas. Flush with the heady success of a two-night run in a seventy-five seat theater on campus, he loped off to New York to seek his fortune, taking the female lead of the play with him. I felt like Nora in "A Doll's House," and was almost ready to meet her fate.

It was Ingrid who helped me snap out of it. She picked flowers for me and generally tried to lift my spirits in her own inimitable style. One day, I came back to the Coop after class and found she had slapped a bumper sticker that said, "A Woman Needs a Man Like a Fish Needs a Bicycle" on my bedroom door. She also brought me fiery feminist tracts about the general lousiness of men and recruited me to work in a local soup kitchen, just to lift my spirits. I'm not sure I agreed with all her sentiments, but at least Ingrid forced me to realize things could be worse: I could have volunteered to work in a soup kitchen regularly. Or, I could have been born a fish.

Naturally, I have felt somewhat indebted to Ingrid for pulling me back from the precipice of Hartley Heartache, though even that ancient gratitude had begun to wear thin. And as soon as Ingrid mentioned the reunion, I slowly shifted from obsessing over her finicky foodism and instead became like Alice in Wonderland, "curiouser and curiouser" to discover what happened to Hartley, Gary, and some of the other alumni. Which of them would actually come to a reunion? I realized one thing: Just in case Hartley or Gary showed up, I wanted to look far more dazzling than dowdy.

Besides, I'd done pretty well for myself, too. I married Jeff after graduate school, and we had produced four children who, by any objective standards, were good-looking and with above average IQs. I'd achieved my goal of becoming a writer, and even had written a couple of books. But did I *look* successful? Would people see me at the reunion and say, "Wow! Judy hasn't aged a bit!" Or would they say, "Gee, too bad she didn't take better care of herself," as they shook their heads sadly and walked away, feeling vaguely superior.

Perhaps, if I allowed Ingrid and her health-consciousness to inspire me, *I* could be the one at the reunion to feel vaguely superior! This could be an opportunity on a silver platter, if only I could muster the fortitude.

"It sounds like a great idea," I said to Ingrid. "A good reason for me to try to finally get in shape before I see old friends again."

Ingrid visibly brightened. "Your own LIFE is a good enough reason for you to get in shape, Judy, but if it takes a reunion to get you going, take ownership of that thought! Maybe you'd like to help me organize it. I'm the reunion co-chair, but I could really use some help with PR and logistics, since I live out of town and the reunion would be here. Only thing is, I just want to be able to plan the menu, if you don't mind."

That figured. I guess we could count on a dinner of organic bok choy and marinated tofu steaks. "Sure, Ingrid. I'll help where I can."

I suppose it's a good thing that Ingrid and I now had the logistics of the reunion to talk about. Otherwise, there might have been little to prevent me from killing her while she remained in my house. She had morphed into a health food harridan, issuing dire warnings about everything I fed my family and myself. At least she wasn't around that much, though, since she couldn't bear to go more than four hours without running off to lift some weights or do a yoga routine in the family room.

As her visit mercifully drew to a close, Ingrid offered to cook dinner for the entire family. A risky proposition, but I didn't want to appear ungracious.

I was exhausted just watching her prepare the meal. She spent the entire afternoon soaking beans, double rinsing barley and pummeling a roll of something called "Betsy's Bulgur Burger" into submission. No wonder her pectorals were so firm.

"Well, dig in!" Ingrid invited as she set the repast down in front of us.

Although I forced down a few bites, my children sat there looking terror-stricken. Finally, my daughter spoke up. "How long are you staying?" she asked Ingrid.

"Oh, I'm leaving tomorrow for a Tae Bo conference in Chicago," she said, swilling a green beverage made of pureed spinach, zucchini and royal bee jelly, "but I've had a great time. Thanks so much for your hospitality!"

Realizing that her leftover whole grains and organic brown rice would probably exceed FAA regulations for allowable weight on the airplane, Ingrid left the remaining groceries from Seven Grain Heaven with us. Anyway, I'm putting it all to good use. Our hamsters love cozying up in their new beds of puffed spelt, and no one would ever guess the treasure trove of vitamins hidden in my steel-cut oat-spackled hallways.

November 10

Well, Ingrid may be gone, but she is not forgotten. Not only did she leave me with a long list of things to do for the reunion, but now other health demons are circling my wagon, one aerobics training circuit at a time. At the Rabbi's Roundtable class today, where I go each week, who should breeze in but Tanya, filling everyone in about her recent weekend at the Oaks, a pricey spa nestled in the outskirts of town. From what I had gathered from Tanya and others who had secluded themselves there, the days revolved around toning and stretching classes, punctuated by leisurely meals of lightly steamed vegetables, served over a discussion of the most optimal methods for colonic irrigation. An exciting night at the Oaks consisted of lying down on a hard, narrow table, wearing only cucumber slices on your eyelids and mud on most other places, and waiting for some solidly built woman named Pia to start kneading your muscles into a coma.

I wondered what had brought Tanya to the Oaks. She was already fit and health-conscious. During the years I had known Tanya, I had never seen her eat sugar. Oh, she had brought boxes of chocolates and other forms of the refined white substance to *me,* as a hostess gift, but personally, she never touched the stuff. I think psychologists call this kind of behavior "passive-aggressive." And though she was already rail thin, her experience at the Oaks put her in Ingrid's league of seeming to have just arrived from the revelation at Sinai.

"I just can't tell you how fabulous I feel! I haven't eaten any white flour or red meat for a month now, and I'm completely off caffeine," Tanya enthused.

"Can it, will ya, Tanya?" I said, protectively stroking my cup of high-octane Columbian roast. "Some of us haven't had our morning ration of Oreos yet." Tanya gave me a look that blended sympathy and condescension in equal measure. The other women in the class reacted to my comment with polite titters, mingled with accusatory silence. I felt ashamed. But really, how much of this could a person take?

"I mean, I'm glad for you, I guess," I stammered, "but it is the holiday season, after all! Some of us are looking forward to festive dinners and parties! There's always January 1!" I said, my smile transparently fake.

Tanya said, "You go ahead and enjoy, but remember, you'll feel fabulous if you can get off the refined flour, sugar, meat, . . ."

"Yeah, yeah, I get the idea," I said, when, to my immense

relief, the rabbi came in to start the class. Given this type of girl talk before we got into the nitty gritty of the story of Abraham and Sarah (who, if I am not mistaken, never had weight problems), I felt pretty shallow.

November 17

I don't see why I should let Ingrid and Tanya get to me like this. Let *them* give birth four times and see if they don't qualify to have the words "Rand-McNally" printed on vast regions of baby-stretched abdomen. And I could do this too, if I really wanted to. The question is, do I really want to?

November 22

Well, perhaps I *ought* to really want to. This became clear to me today when I went shopping for some holiday clothes, using a gift card that Jeff had given me a while back. While trying on an A-line gray skirt and tasseled sweater, I poked my head out of the dressing room to find Maria, my saleslady, for her opinion. She was nearby, so I stepped out to show her how I looked.

Maria then did something that she lived to regret just seconds later. She gently pushed me toward the three-way mirror and said, "Here, let's see how you look from all sides." Immediately, I threw myself against the mirror, as if trying to shelter a small child from falling debris, and shrieked, "Are you nuts? One mirror is quite enough, Maria!" Maria backed away, a bit frightened, and said in a soothing tone, the kind often reserved for speaking to the criminally insane, "Of course. Whatever you say. The outfit does look lovely, though."

What's wrong with me? As if I don't know! Fifteen lousy pounds are making me deranged. The same fifteen pounds I have been trying to lose since the Bush (The Elder) administration. I'm not an entirely hopeless case. After all, I have lost ten pounds already, but it has taken me five years! At this rate, I'll be absolutely svelte by the time I hit the shuffleboard courts at the old age home where on Wednesdays they'll put me on a bus and take me to an aquarium or to a concert, where I will no longer be able to hear the music. But who wants to wait that long? I need to get a grip and lose this featherbedding once and for all. Even taking the slow boat to China method of weight loss, I should be able to lose the weight easily before the reunion in June. Besides, with the reunion just a few days after my birthday, I could give myself the gift of a glorious figure! If Ingrid can do it, and if Tanya can catapult herself into the stratosphere of energy and robust health, I will, too!

I'm glad I bought the outfit, and a pair of jeans, too, in my current size, not my hoped-for size, since I wanted to walk and breathe at the same time. I may not have attained weight perfection yet, but at least I'm entitled to some new duds. I'm slowly, ever so slowly, gaining courage to begin a diet again. Just not before I polish off that pan of Duncan Hines brownies. I hate to see perfectly good food go to waste.

November 23

At home, I caused quite a stir by my startling appearance in jeans, an event as rare as a sighting of Halley's comet. After all, I hadn't even worn pants other than pajamas since 1987. This predates the birth of any of my kids and therefore explains their shock. What was stodgy old Mom doing in a get-up like this?

They all about fell on their faces when they came home from school and saw me. My daughter, who at seven years old is always in the midst of animated conversation, even when alone, trailed off mid-sentence after sweeping me up with one horrified glance. She swallowed hard, and, perhaps for the first time in her existence, was speechless.

I asked her what she thought of Mommy's new look, and she said, "You're not going to wear these *out of the house*, are you?" When I just smiled mysteriously, she apparently saw her entire future social life flash before her eyes and shouted anxiously, "I want the truth!"

Even my eldest son, whose idea of high-class behavior is using cutlery, was too polite to comment. He glanced at my denim-clad legs and looked away, the way people do when faced with the abnormal or the disfigured. The other boys, as they always do after school, saw nothing until they were knee-deep in the pantry, on a search-and-destroy mission. If I had been wearing a toga made of aluminum foil, they probably wouldn't have noticed as long as we still had Chips Ahoy in the house.

But I was amused. They don't know that I'm on a mission! I will get in shape! I will transform before their eight eyes into New Mom! Lean and Healthy Mom! Fashion-Daring Mom! One day they'll come home and see me in single-digit jeans, looking about as hot as a post-forty-year-old mom can look, given that she has not had the benefit of liposuction or chemical peels. So what if I have made this same resolution hundreds of times already? This time I mean it! I'll show them.

November 25

While cleaning up the family room today, I came across some old magazines and flipped through them to see which ones were worth keeping. One immediately caught my eye with its promise of a quiz posing the question: "How fit are you?" I suspected that I already knew the answer. Still, I sat down with the magazine and a pen and took the quiz, hoping it might help motivate me to begin my new diet and exercise routine. Here's what it asked:

1. You believe you would be more fit . . .
a. If you lost ten pounds

b. If you could run from the house to the car without feel
ing you needed to call the paramedics

c. If you were Meg Ryan

2. Which of the following actions can you do?

a. Bend back far enough to look at the wall behind you

b. Perform ten strong push-ups

c. Beat twenty other people to the register at the
Nordstrom semi-annual women's wear sale

d. Think about exercise for five minutes before
needing to lie down

3. Your favorite kind of sport is. . .

a. Rollerblading in the park

b. Rock climbing

c. Mall walking

d. Computer chess

4. Your idea of portion control is. . .

a. Using a measuring cup when serving yourself food,
being careful not to exceed a predetermined number
of calories or carbohydrates

b. Thinking about your hunger and listening to what your
body says it really wants to eat

c. Forcing extravagant servings onto the plates of your thin
friends and relatives when they are guests for dinner

d. Something airlines do to annoy passengers

5. You can do aerobic activity, such as running, bicycling, or speed walking. . .

a. Six times a week for at least twenty minutes

b. Three times weekly for fifteen minutes

c. About once a week, for about eight minutes

d. When someone points a gun to your feet and shouts,
"Dance!"

6. Which of the following leaves you out of breath the fastest?
a. Jogging two miles
b. Gardening
c. Doing the dishes
d. Hearing the words, "Dessert is served!"

7. You weight train at least three days a week
a. True
b. Damnable lie

8. Which would you say most accurately describes your fitness level?
a. Eligible to run the Boston Marathon
b. Can complete a five-mile walkathon
c. Can drive the Boston Marathon
d. Able to grab the TV remote and channel surf without getting winded during the Boston Marathon

I tallied my score, somehow earning a negative number. The magazine interpreted this result as follows: "Apparent hostility to exercise and preoccupation with food may worsen your health, which is already questionable. Introducing modest changes, such as walking for fifteen minutes after meals, can only enhance your otherwise pathetic health profile."

Well, this was a sobering wake-up call! In the same magazine, another article discussed the surging demand for plus-sized clothing throughout the nation. This was one trend I did not want to join. After finishing my cleaning, and dumping the magazine, I dusted off my tennis shoes and walked for a half-hour around the neighborhood. Once outside, I noticed that it was, indeed, a beautiful day.

DECEMBER

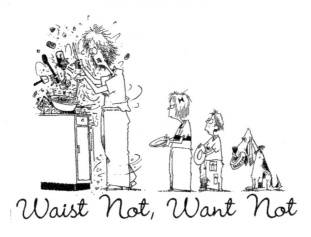

Waist Not, Want Not

December 1

Of course, sticking to this kind of resolution isn't easy, especially at holiday time. Tonight we all celebrated Grandma's ninety-third birthday, and came back stuffed fuller than a new down pillow. Our family's favorite party platter is a cholesterol-fest of deli meats, potato salad, cole slaw, and enough rye and egg bread to feed at least two NFL teams. I believe I showed admirable restraint, passing up the cake – chocolate cake! Otherwise, everyone ate with abandon, except for poor Chloe, whose pancreas was acting up again. She made a pathetic show of it, desperate to eat along with the rest of us.

"Down, Chloe, down!" shouted my sister-in-law Brenda, diligent caretaker of this tiny four-legged foundling, as the canine kept leaping up onto the table, trying to cop some licks of corned beef and mayonnaise. Brenda remained alert to any clandestine deli deliveries to Chloe under the table, and even accused the birthday girl herself of slipping a finger's worth of roast beef to the dog. "No food for Chloe, Gran!"

"Nah! Nah! I know already!" said Gran in an accent about

as charming as German could ever sound. "I didn't gif her nutting!" Even at her age, Grandma looks so good and has such beautiful skin that men still sometimes make passes at her. Last week at the cardiologist's office, a dapper gentleman looked at her admiringly and said, "If only I was a few years younger, I'd ask you out." He was eighty-eight. Gran's doctor has even laid odds on her living to 100. I wondered if Gran had some health secrets I should know about. I sidled over to her, and asked her if she attended any of the exercise classes offered at the upscale retirement home where she lives.

Grandma laughed. "Me? I am too lazy!" she said.

"Did you ever used to exercise?"

Her answer stung me. "I never exercised a day in my life!" she said. "Only taking care of my house, dat's the only exercise I ever did!" Well, not exactly. Grandma never learned to drive, and until her mid-eighties she still walked to the grocery store, carting her things home in a small rolling basket. And I know for a fact that in her room, Gran keeps a stash of chocolates, and dips into them without guilt. When we come to visit, Gran likes to play the hostess. With effort, she gets up from her chair and offers us apples, bananas, and, from a private drawer that she opens with a key, her lovely assortment of all kinds of chocolates. Perhaps this, then, is part of her secret.

I wish I had Grandma's total nonchalance when it comes to food, but instead, I am always calculating calories, fat grams, and cholesterol. Of course, at Gran's age she eats very little, and protests "Ach! Too much!" before anyone can finish dropping a tablespoon of potatoes on her plate, but I suspect that even in her salad days, Gran simply ate what she wanted, when she wanted, and never calculated a single caloric intake in nearly a century!

I can't count on having her good luck. Besides, she's Jeff's grandmother, not mine, so I can't even claim any of her DNA. But old age, despite its problems, sounds a sight better to me than not getting there at all. Even at my age, I'm starting to believe that my knees, which are making funny creaking noises, might benefit from an occasional shot of WD-40.

Maybe tomorrow I'll muster the courage to get on the scale.

December 3

The calendar is closing in on me. December already! Where did the year go? And why, in the last year, have I lost just about everything I own except some weight? I've lost my keys, my sunglasses, and my peace of mind. I've lost my wallet, eight library books, and even, for a heart-stopping half-hour at an outdoor fair, one of the kids. I seem to be able to lose everything except this padding.

Just as a reminder of this fact, today's spam e-mails were nearly all insulting in nature. One e-mailer invited me out on a date, if I could meet him in Sydney, Australia. The next suggested, with no subtlety whatsoever, that I start "loosing" weight — today! Do people who can't even spell correctly expect me to cough up money for their charlatan plans? Besides, my weight already *is* "loose!" Then I received an exclusive offer to purchase an Apple Cider Vinegar potion for only sixteen dollars and ninety-five cents, but I've already got apple cider vinegar at home that, if I am not mistaken, only cost me about a buck-sixty-nine.

Since the world is full of scams, I've ruled out the following types of diets and schemes:

1. Any program that has to advertise by stapling flyers on telephone poles.
2. Any product or plan where the ads have misspelled words.
3. Anyone who wants to pay me as a subject in a test to eat a funny fiber-rich candy bar for lunch for the next thirty days.
4. Any potion, powder or swill promising to make people begin confusing my body with Pamela Anderson's.

5. Any program that costs more than my monthly car payment.
6. Any program demanding I buy their meals, have group encounter sessions, or perform unnatural acts of multilevel marketing.

I'm sure the list will grow, but so far, I think this is a good start.

December 5

This morning I had my regular visit with Dr. Charles, who helps me with my creaking spine. While I was lying down on the table, waiting for him to whack my vertebrae back in line, I asked his advice about getting fit. His face turned serious, and he crossed his muscular arms. "Do you eat sugar?" he asked.

Never ask for diet advice from someone who openly admits to doing 250 sit-ups a day and drinks spirulina juice for breakfast. "Sugar is my lifeline to sanity," I confessed.

Dr. Charles then launched into a lecture about the evils of refined sugar, and its devastating impact over time on my pancreas. Shades of Ingrid, haunting me like the ghost of Macbeth! He also said that sugar depressed my immune system, and here I thought that it was lack of sugar that depressed my entire soul!

"Sugar makes it harder for you to recover from colds and flu, and if you don't want to end up in a diabetic coma one day, cut it out!" he implored.

This sounded rather harsh to me. Did I really eat too much sugar? I considered whether he could be right. Obviously I ate sweets on special occasions: my birthday, my kids' birthdays, and also those of my husband, first cousins, second cousins, second cousins once removed, friends, and anyone else reported on the Today Show as marking that special day. Sometimes it occurred to me that, somewhere in the world, some lonely person was having a birthday and yet no one was taking her to lunch. It only seemed right that I have a cookie or piece of pie in solidarity, beaming my own personal happy birthday signals across the miles, letting this poor soul know that at least I had not forgotten. Then of course there were other special times, such as anniversaries, staff office parties (wherever they may be), National PMS Stress Day, and Military Appreciation Week.

And, obviously, there were religious observances, national holidays, and other inherently happy days, such as the first day of spring, Freedom from Tax Day, and Barbershop Quartet Day. Was that excessive?

Frankly, Dr. Charles wasn't the first to tell me to knock out an entire beloved food group from my life. Years before, I had gone to Dr. Li, a tiny Vietnamese acupuncturist who helped me with a tough pregnancy. She made me stick out my tongue and examined it with disapproving eyes. "You eat cheese!" she accused, having somehow divined this information from her look at my tongue. When I admitted that I loved cheese, I discovered that Dr. Li was very excitable. She started pacing around in an agitated state, shouting, "Never! Never eat cheese! Never again in your life!!!!" Did they worship dairy products in Vietnam? If so, it would account for her state of distress. Her office was plastered with signed posters from Sylvester Stallone, arguably a more famous patient than me. Did Rambo need permission from this diminutive doctor to eat fettuccine Alfredo? I doubted it.

Dr. Li's standard diet advice to everyone she met, no matter if they had come with gastric problems or a shin splint, was to eat chicken soup for dinner every night with brown rice and vegetables on the side. Every night! With visions of Dr. Li flailing her acupuncture needle-laden arms around the room, I was chastened to lard my lasagnas with fewer layers of cheese than I used to, and I even experimented with fat-free cheese, a substance that had the consistency and taste of rubber cement. I decided to meet Dr. Li halfway and go with low-fat cheese. Of course, I never told her I continued to poison my system in this way.

I left Dr. Charles' office with my back feeing a lot better, but my psyche further pummeled. If all these other folks could muster self-discipline, I could too. With New Year's coming up soon, I'm going to get this right, once and for all.

December 6

The question is, what weight-loss plan should I choose to begin my path to slimness? This is no easy task. At last count, there were more diets on the market than there are dollars in the federal deficit. In the last few days, I poured over several diet books from the library, including these:

The Pineapple Principle — Every meal starts with pineapple and ends with hot chile peppers and mustard. The combination of these "thermogenic" foods is supposed to scare the metabolism nearly to death, which makes it burn fat quickly.

Protein A'Plenty Planet — Bacon and eggs for breakfast, chicken (with skin) or beef for lunch and dinner. A half a cup of broccoli or other green vegetable is allowed every other Tuesday. Fridays are "free" days and therefore you can have radishes and an eighth of a cantaloupe. Theory: the protein builds muscle, while the elimination of joy in eating depresses the appetite.

Hollywood Celeb Special Effects Diet Beverage — Based on a sample population of several thousand Hollywood extras, this diet consists of guzzling a concentrated, glow-in-the-dark vitamin-enriched drink that substitutes for a chewable meal. Add water, shake, and drink up! Time saved by not eating allows more time to work out. Endorsed by an aging B-movie star whom I vaguely remember from the days of carbon paper, this gambit has limited appeal, especially since the ingredients are mostly concentrated fruit juice, but cost twenty times the price of the real thing.

My Body, My Life — Wildly popular book written by a college dropout, this plan calls for eight small snacks a day, so as to keep the metabolism humming at a steady pace. The drawback: each snack must be nutritionally calibrated so as to have exactly 42.7 percent protein, 39.1 percent carbohydrates, and 18.2 percent fat. Even tiny variations in this formula will throw the whole thing into disarray. Because it is tricky to maintain the right composition of foods, the author sells shake mixes, protein bars and other prepared snacks that take the guesswork out of eating and any available discretionary income out of the wallet. When not snacking, dieters need to either weight train or perform twenty-minute aerobic sprints.

Writer's Cramp Your Way To Thinness – A plan based on journaling for five hours per day about every aspect of eating: what you plan to eat, when you plan to eat it, emotional "triggers" that make you think about eating, how many times you chew before swallowing each bite and the emotional reactions you have to each mastication cycle, how much you enjoyed your food, and other feelings associated with food choices, your mother, and your long-distance phone company. The theory: devoting all this time to writing leaves time for only one meal a day.

If You Lived On Okinawa, You'd Be Thin, Too – Based on research of eighty-seven centenarians living on Okinawa who do little except drink tea, garden, and repeat the mantra, "Hara hachi bu," which means, "Enough rice already! It's time for Tai Chi!" I also started saying "Hara hachi bu!" at dinner to remind me to stop eating, but it didn't work. However, it did train the kids to say "Gesundtheit!" at regular intervals and make them get up to bring me tissues.

Bad Carbohydrates and the Women Who Love Them – Similar to *Protein A' Plenty Planet*, this diet shuns carbohydrates and explains why women who allow carbohydrates to control their lives are probably destined never to marry. Includes success stories from women who found freedom from rice and grains and, even if they never married, at least snagged live-in boyfriends.

The Happy Hour Scarfsdale Diet – Unlike the other carbo-hating regimens, this plan allows dieters to eat as many carbohydrates as they wish, provided they are all eaten in one hour or less a day. I know a married couple who tried this diet as a tag team. But when I invited them over one night for what I hoped would be a leisurely dinner with us, they kept looking at their watches, asking impatiently when dessert would be served. Personally, entertaining is hard enough without this added pressure.

I considered each of these books and their recommendations, then promptly rejected them. Not only do I hate anything that smacks of regimentation, I once tried Tai Chi and found it induced a state of catatonic boredom. I also hate mustard and am allergic to cayenne pepper. Instead, I am going to get in shape and lose weight with a program of my own devising. I will call it, "Chew Less, Move More," a name that aptly sums up the premise. I'll cut way down on white flour, sugar and fat, and eat more low-calorie and vegetable-based foods. I will make exercise a priority, and see how it goes! If it succeeds, perhaps I'll figure out a way to stretch the four words of the title into a 250-page book and finally move that annoying Dr. Atkins off the bestseller list.

December 7

My old bathroom scale, the one I bought for seven bucks about fifteen years ago, says that everybody weighs sixty-eight pounds, so I realized the time had come to chuck it and get a real one. I went to Target, the place I go to save money but always end up realizing there are about 100 other things I need once I'm there.

I wanted to make the easy decision first, so I asked a store clerk where I would find a measuring tape. But nothing is that simple. He took me a half-mile away to the district of home and gardening supplies, and handed me a metalized measuring tape the size of a garden hose! I looked at him in absolute horror. How dare he insult me like that! Then I realized that he didn't know what the heck I wanted it for, and just assumed I needed to measure the living room for new carpet, and not my hips and waist. I then told him I wanted the kind of measuring tape used for sewing, and then I walked back another half-mile to the section of notions.

Measuring tape in hand, I then went on a hunt for a good bathroom scale. All I can say is that at least one of these scale manufacturers needs a new marketing plan, because calling a bathroom scale the "Up-Scale" is pretty slack witted. I want to *down*scale, if you please, so I didn't even examine the Up-Scale's other features. The "Autobahn" scale had a sleek design, but I didn't see why I needed anything with racing stripes and a 120 kilometer-per-hour capacity. I did not need the "heavy gauge, extra-wide platform" either.

I finally chose the "Thinner" scale, since the name sounded appropriately optimistic. It had a 300-pound capacity, which meant several of the kids could jump up and down on it all at once without breaking it, and it also had a non-skid surface, in case I was in a crazy "Autobahn" kind of mood and felt like careening toward it to get weighed. It's digital and therefore cheat-proof, since I can't tinker with a dial or adjust the "zero" mark in a way that would be favorable to me. On this scale, I have to touch a keypad in the middle to activate it, as if I am touching some special oracle. Then it shows me a bunch of 888's followed by a zero, after which I get on, trying not to make skid marks. It is also guaranteed for ten years or 10,000 pounds, whichever comes first.

December 8

I went to get my fat tested today. It came back positive. I cannot say that this came as a total surprise. But if I am going to get serious about lowering my weight and boosting my health, I need to face the cold, hard, brutal, nauseating facts. Figuring out how fat I really was has been on my "to do" list for about five years, but when I finally screwed up the courage to try to get an answer, I realized the job was too complicated for me.

Here is the "simple" calculation for figuring out the "body mass index," or BMI. The BMI is the number that many nutritional and government experts use to decide if someone is too heavy or not. I took the formula from one of the many diet books now sitting like a millstone on the bookshelf in my office. It goes like this:

Weight in kilograms divided by height in meters squared (kg)/ht (m)2, multiplied by shoe size, divided by number of shoes in your closet, squared by income tax bracket.

This was no help to me at all. My formal education did not prepare me for life in the metric system. However, I could also try to figure out my BMI the old-fashioned way:

Weight in pounds divided by height in inches squared, multiplied by 703, multiplied by dress size, divided by number of recent parking tickets, squared by number of recently discovered endangered species. Now, according to the government, a healthy BMI is supposed to be between nineteen and twenty-five, so I don't know how I came up with the number of 42,598%, but then again, math has never been my forte.

As luck would have it, though, the day I failed to correctly calculate my BMI I also received a coupon in the mail for fifteen bucks off a procedure that would answer this nagging question in a highly scientific fashion, with no math skills needed from me. I drove right over to Flab-No-More!, a nutrition counseling center conveniently located next to Muscle Mart, "the Mecca for the muscle-building mentality." I had planned to check out Muscle Mart after I heard the awful truth about my own body composition.

When Sydney asked me to get on the scale, I had a sick feeling in my stomach. Usually, in preparation for a Serious Weigh-In, I cut my nails, shave my legs, scrub with a loofa, get a haircut, starve for two days and wear a skimpy cotton dress that weighs less than a letter-sized envelope. I had neglected to do any of these things. Still, although dressed like an Eskimo in

February, I kept my head held high while I stepped on the scale. Even here, in my private diary, I will not disclose my true weight, but will only say that it is a number with three figures, which starts with a "1" and ends in a "4.6." Sydney, bless her skinny little heart, took pity and deducted two whole pounds – one for clothing and the other for good sportsmanship.

We next moved on to the nub of the biscuit. She took out calipers the size of ice tongs and pinched me in several private areas, jotting down numbers as she went along. I felt utterly humiliated. I had leftovers in my freezer that weighed more than Sydney. In any case, the deed was soon done. The good news is that I have nearly 100 pounds of lean body mass. The "other" news is that the rest is, well, *fat*. Sydney's office was festooned with "before" and "after" photos of people who had become warriors in the fight against flab. In a remarkable coincidence, each "before" photo showed the woman or man appearing clinically depressed, even if he or she hadn't been heavy to begin with. This may be accounted for by the fact that all were trussed in ill-fitting bathing suits and told to slouch their shoulders at forty-five degree angles. Droopy hips and tummies were only matched by equally droopy expressions. Adding insult to injury, some of these poor dejected souls were photographed from the back, so as to show them at full disadvantage. The "after" photos showed the most fantastic transformations imaginable, especially considering that they had happened in only six weeks. The formerly thick-waisted were now all sinew and gristle, topped by beaming, tanned faces with smirky little smiles, as if they had not only lost weight, but also found some charming little tax shelter in the Bahama Islands. The women wore skimpy bikinis the size of two rubber bands, stiletto heels, and daringly red nail polish.

To her credit, Sydney told me not to worry about my weight, because muscle weighs more than fat, and often, people will end up weighing MORE after getting fit than they did before. Just what I wanted to hear: the probability that even getting in shape would add pounds to my short, matronly frame!

I thanked her for her time, and soldiered on to Muscle Mart. This was one scary place. Even to look around I had to sign a waiver indemnifying them for any injuries I might incur "resulting in complete or partial paralysis, heart attacks, serious spinal injuries, dismemberment or even death." The potential risks associated with visiting Muscle Mart got worse from there, but I got the general idea. When I looked around this manic muscle meat market, I understood why their attorneys had written that waiver. First, I was nearly dismembered just walking too close to a seventy-pound bar clanging down on one of the weight machines. Then, with my poor heart already racing, I thought I'd have a coronary just watching these guys and gals grimacing with extraordinary effort just to inflate muscles that were already more pumped than anything I had ever seen outside of a cartoon. Most of the men had built such gargantuan pectorals that their elbows were suspended in different area codes. Muscle Mart was about the size of Rhode Island, and all I heard were the sounds of banging weights, pulleys slamming down, and grunting. The smallest hand weights I saw were the size of small car tires and must have weighed about forty-five pounds each. One puckish little man jumped an invisible jump rope all the way from a Nautilus machine to the men's room. A calorie burned is a calorie earned.

Upstairs, another guy was chugging water out of a keg. No wimpy little half-liter bottles for him. A personal trainer pressed his hands against the feet of a man attempting some kind of bizarre physical contortion. Mostly, I saw a lot of men straining so hard to lift weights they bore expressions that in my opinion should only be seen on women in labor. At Muscle Mart, no area of the anatomy was too obscure for physical fitness. I saw one guy take something that looked like a leather harness with a chain attached and strap it on his head, as if he were waiting for someone to take him for a walk. I wondered what in God's name he would do with this, when, to my amazement, he attached a huge metal discus to the chain, and practiced lifting it with his head, veins bulging from his neck. And these people were paying for this! By this point, I had pretty much ruled out Muscle Mart as an appropriate venue for my own physical development. I continued to walk the gym's vast acreage, working up a spanking appetite. Then I went out for a tuna sandwich, easy on the mayo.

December 10

I found a book called *Facing Your Inner Buddha*, and followed its instructions to look at myself in the mirror, attired only in the get-up the good Lord had given me. As I undressed, I heard the soundtrack from some really horrid scary movie playing in my mind, the kind of music that tells you that the young, innocent, beautiful woman relaxing in bed, sipping a nice cup of herbal tea and reading a scholarly book about the history of French classical composers, is about to have an ax murderer smash in her windows and then do unspeakable things to her.

I waited till the afternoon light had faded a bit, so as to make the effect of my facing myself less traumatic. It didn't help. I stood before the mirror, eyes closed. I opened them very slowly. When I saw my reflection, it signaled my brain to continue playing the soundtrack from the scary movie, the part where the scream of high-pitched violins lets you know that the ax murderer is in the house.

Now that I faced both my inner and outer Buddhas in the unvarnished daylight, I resolved never to eat another carbohydrate again in my life. Time to change this music!

December 14

Well, it's been four whole days and I don't seem to have much to show for my new conviction to lose weight. In fact, I have managed to lose only one ounce, which may be accounted for by a new haircut. Anyway, with the holiday season and all, it's going to take a lot more effort than I've put into this so far, which, basically, has been looking pensive for a few minutes a day while I beam instructions to my metabolism to try to make it understand that burning calories is not a spectator sport. And, even though today happens to be Thailand Constitution Day and would have been Dorothy Lamour's birthday, I am celebrating in spirit only. No fatty foods will pass my lips, despite these festive occasions.

I can't say I've made absolutely no progress, since I went to the library and checked out several other diet books. As with the first batch of books, however, I have been busily rejecting one after the other.

Today I gave the old heave-ho to *Daily Detox Drills*, a 300-page book that devotes the first 260 pages to scaring the daylights out of you about the imminent collapse of all your internal organs. The author, a naturopathic physician who had his author photo taken while dangling from a tree, claims that pretty much everything in Western society is poisoning us all with horrid toxins that make it darned near impossible for our livers and kidneys to do their 497 different jobs. He claims that not only non-organic foods, but also all manner of household cleansing agents, office supplies, *including correction fluid,* and even certain kinds of mattress pads, make us vulnerable to getting vile intestinal disorders, not to mention PMS (even men!).

I admit, he had me going there for a while, and I just about felt compelled to turn over my laundry detergent to the Department of Defense, convinced it was a bioterrorist weapon, until I got to page 227. That's when we got to the kernel: For optimum health, we need to detoxify our systems, mainly, I learned, through fasting on organic juices and herbal teas. "We must all be ready to make sacrifices for our health," the doc wrote, and I wasn't happy to learn that first on the list of sacrifices were charbroiled burgers, which harbor bacteria that the GI tract, in a cruel twist of fate for the beef industry, converts to carcinogens. The book also got me worried about my "process of elimination." Compared to ideal measures, mine was, in his words, "sluggish." I resolved again to drink more water. I began to feel sorry for my liver, which apparently is a busier appliance than I had ever realized.

I sure like the idea of having a healthier body, better skin color, and a well-oiled internal system. But if I did this detoxification program, I would need to do something much harder than give up charbroiled burgers. I'd need to clear my calendar for at least three days so I could stay in bed, think positive thoughts (so as to remove toxic stress from my life) and fast on the juices, pure water and herbal teas. Of course, attaining optimal health has its costs. The author predicted that during this process, I could expect most of the following side effects: bad breath, irritability, offensive body odor, migraines, round-the-clock hunger, muscle aches, and flatulence. Therefore, he recommended that practitioners avoid anything stressful during this time, such as attending Tupperware parties and other prominent social gatherings. What a hoot! What mother with kids at home can manage to clear three whole hours, let alone three days? I could just imagine laying in bed, sipping my tea, windows open, and having one or more kids barge in and remind me it was time for dinner, and what *was* for dinner, anyway? I'd just say, "Sorry, dears, I'm detoxifying. Come back on Thursday."

December 21

That stupid book has now made me paranoid about my liver. Because the last thing I need on my conscious is an unhappy liver, I haven't had a charbroiled burger since reading *Daily Detox Drills*. I had to fight off strong cravings on four separate occasions.

And since I now feel really sorry for this poor, beleaguered internal organ, I have also begun making the supreme sacrifice of taking the skin off my chicken. This hasn't been easy. I grew up in a family where we were never allowed to give chicken skin to the dog, since it wasn't good for *her* system, but apparently it was good enough for our pipes. Anyone who turned his or her head at the wrong moment during mealtime in our family was likely to have had the chicken skin speared off his or her plate and onto someone else's. It does make sense that eating something that rubbery cannot possibly be good for you, and I am trying to make peace with life without this fowl overlay.

December 25

Well, it may be Christmas time in the city, but I still have many Chanukah latkes to burn off from last week. After my narrow escape with heart failure during my visit to Muscle Mart, I knew I'd have to ease my way to fitness in the privacy of my own home. Mostly, this is because I refuse to be seen in public in spandex. I borrowed a Richard Simmons video from a friend, and popped it in the VCR. I immediately saw that even now, years after he found his niche catering to the plus-sized crowd, Richard had lost none of his flair. Although most other exercise videos I've seen have fancy or exotic sets, any such gimmicks or other special effects would have been superfluous here: Richard himself was the main event. Wearing his signature steel wool hairstyle, red and white striped shorts (rather too short for good taste, in my opinion) and red tank top glittering with an explosion of starburst sequins, such as you might expect to see on a Rockette at Radio City Music Hall, Richard led his hefty harem in twenty minutes of lowish impact aerobics. Like an old MGM musical, he broke into song at regular intervals.

He was the most earnest looking fitness instructor I've ever seen, even tearing up during moments of great emotional aerobic impact. Was he ever proud of his girls, hustling their Hadassah hips down to more humble proportions! Richard seemed to like everything he said so much that he repeated it, with emphasis: "Oh, I believe in you, BELIEVE IN YOU!" he shouted, shimmying and sashaying across the floor. "Are you on your toes? YOUR TOES?" Richard's students looked deliriously happy, and my guess is that in a society that even has to ask the question, "Is Gwynneth Paltrow too thin?" these gals were grateful not to be the token tubbies on screen. They were, in fact, the *raison d'etre* of the video. The atmosphere was part Salsa-disco, part church revival meeting, as the energetic ladies, and one token guy other than Richard, whooped, yelped, and otherwise proved their enthusiasm for the blintz-shaped patron saint of the padded set. They clearly loved him, or at least were paid to look as if they did. I felt alarmed that I couldn't quite keep up even with the heftiest Hollys on the video. Those babes, even the 250-pounders, could really shimmy and strut. And I admired their professionally applied make-up – a sure sight better than my own!

I had to turn away and blush when Richard tossed off some of his "come-hither" looks from the TV, using cheap come-on lines in a variety of accents. These accents changed with no prior warning. "Come OVAH to me!" (British) and "I hope you're feeling hot, I HOPE YOU'RE FEELING HOT!" (American singles bar), alarming things that would have earned him a good slap in the face had he said them in person and had I been more fully clothed. During a John Travolta "Saturday Night Fever" move, while we were all jabbing fingers heavenward and strutting along, I felt the spirit move me. Richard believed in me, BELIEVED IN ME! If this wide world of women could have lost anywhere from thirty-five to more than 125 pounds, which they in fact did, as it said on the video, I could surely lose fifteen, FIFTEEN!

As Richard sashayed into a Latin rumba move, asking me, "Are you feeling it, FEELING IT?" with a suspicious Julio Iglesias accent, I couldn't help myself any longer. Although temporarily blinded by his sequined get-up, I shouted to the television, "Yes, Richard, I'm FEELING IT! BELIEVE IN ME!" One of my kids, spying on me through a crack in the door, suddenly ran in fear down the hall and into a sibling's room, which was just as well, as Richard and I were now doing some kind of Egyptian Nephrititi-type dance, with Richard reminding me again that he BELIEVED IN ME!

Before I knew it, we were cooling down. In a whispery voice, Richard told me how proud of me he was, HOW PROUD! We cooled down while making "butterfly arms" to help us fly free, and then, just like that, it ended. We were MAGNIFICO! It had to be true; Richard said so. But even with all Richard's oleaginous praise, the fact is, I was out of breath, and not because of any of Richard's brazenly flirtatious lines, or even the sequins.

December 26

I noted on my calendar that today is National Whiner's Day as well as Slovenia Independence Day, but I resisted my old habit of using sugar-smacked food to celebrate. Reluctantly, I passed up the last cinnamon bun we had in the house. Instead, I tried to absorb the message of a new video called *Subliminal Thinness* that I found at the library. The video intrigued me because everything I have been reading about exercise says that boredom can really sabotage your plan to get in shape. It was also intriguing because it had absolutely no cover graphic. I suppose even *that* was subliminal. The gist was that by "hearing" and "seeing" the subliminal messages on screen, and watching the video over a period of thirty days, I might begin to feel, act and be thinner, *effortlessly!* The entire video consisted of four rotating camera shots of a lakefront, with waves lapping gently against the rocks or the shore. At the beginning, I, the viewer, read a list of the messages I would continue to get while watching the video, such as "I have self-discipline," "I will eat, think and act thin," and "I never really liked crème brulee, anyway."

However, I remain skeptical of the split-second flashes of

the subliminal messages themselves. After all, how can I be sure that the message beamed for a nanosecond really said, "I am determined to drink eight glasses of water a day" rather than "You chowderhead! Only a nitwit would sit there watching this tripe!" I did listen hard for the subliminal messages that they said would be barely audible under the sounds of the waves, but I only heard the sound of my stomach rumbling. I'm not sure what happened at the end of the tape, since the sounds of those gentle waves put me to sleep. In my dreams, I saw visions of subliminal tiramisu. The kind that makes you drool.

December 28

This morning I called a fitness instructor recommended by Dr. Charles. Ready to cash in on other overfed individuals making their umpteenth New Year's resolutions to trim down, "GI Joe Jerome" is running a New Year's special: Do fifty push-ups with him in the morning by the beach, get the second fifty for free! Dr. Charles told me that he personally trains with Jerome, but wasn't sure if he really had been in the military. "All I know is, when he says, run, we run!" Dr. Charles said.

GI Joe Jerome had a kind of "Make my day" tone of voice. "Yo," he answered, his voice about eight octaves lower than baritone. When I asked him about his qualifications, he said, "I'm a world-champion in bare-knuckle fights, you know, the kind you see on pay-per-view, that kinda thang," he said. I tried to convey my deep disappointment that his classes didn't meet my schedule. Although next time I need to learn some bare-knuckle fighting techniques, I'd certainly know whom to call.

Later in the day, my prospects improved. On my way to the library, I saw a car advertising something called "Boot Camp Fitness." I hadn't particularly been shopping for military-style training, but as long as the program didn't promise pay-per-view-style wrestling, I was open to the suggestion.

When I got home, I called and spoke to the Major. He was

the real enchilada, a bona fide United States Air Force veteran and now a personal fitness trainer helping the less-than-beautiful people of Los Angeles peel off pounds. I just read, in fact, that there are about 88,000 personal fitness trainers in the entire United States. My guess is that 87,000 of them are right here in Los Angeles. Next to aspiring actors and screenwriters, L.A. must have the highest per-capita population of personal trainers in the solar system.

When the Major told me that he was also a paramedic, I immediately offered up my credit card number. I liked this qualification in an exercise instructor, considering that I've done little more strenuous in the last six months than to wrestle a screaming child into the dentist's chair for a cleaning and hoist a fifteen-pound brisket from the oven. The Major promised to send me a copy of rules for all New Recruits and my Report for Duty Papers, which I will need to sign and return before class, which starts January 7. Boot Camp meets three times a week, rain or shine, and unexcused absences mean that the other recruits in the unit have to do twenty extra push-ups, so attendance will be pretty important to keep up my social standing with the group.

My heart sank when I heard the only times for Boot Camp were six a.m. and again at six p.m., neither particularly family-friendly times. But I liked the Major, and sensed that only a man with actual combat experience would succeed in getting me to move my fanny. So, given a choice between bolting out of bed during deep REM mode and cutting out while the kids were arguing over who sets the table, the choice was easy.

Boot Camp, here I come!

December 31

Today I was overcome by a desire for frozen yogurt. Well, truthfully, I pined for a schooner full of brownie ripple ice cream with hot fudge and heavily blanketed with whipped cream, but I was determined to show self-restraint. Since all the news about dairy products is wildly contradictory, who can blame for me for indulging?

Just today I heard a report on the radio about a new study linking increased consumption of healthy dairy products with a lower risk of getting diabetes and other diseases. But later, I opened up one of my new library books, called *Why Dairy Products Will Kill You!* This book claims that dairy products actually *cause* osteoporosis as well as nearly every ill that plagues the planet, ranging from obesity and allergies to global warming and social snobbery. To prove his thesis that dairy products kill, the author noted that every single person who has ever drunk milk throughout history has died. He also predicted a similar fate for anyone still alive and foolhardy enough to consume dairy. This sounds nutty enough to have been penned by somebody like Dr. Li. Perhaps she writes under a pseudonym?

Truth is, I *have* been avoiding a lot of dairy, but today, on the eve of my new health regimen, I didn't see any harm in a little cup of frozen yogurt.

Was it my fault that the only Baskin-Robbins on my route to pick up the kids from school didn't offer yogurt? As soon as I walked in and realized this, I told myself to walk out, immediately! As usual, I ignored my better instincts and joined a long line, giving me ample time to decide if I wanted a cup of their sugar-free ice cream instead. That wouldn't be so bad. I stood there, debating. I really didn't like their sugar-free ice cream. It left a yucky aftertaste in the mouth. Because I had been fairly restrained dietetically, I hadn't known that the Flavor of the Month, for which this was the very last day, was an obscenely rich swirl of chocolate, brownies, vanilla and mocha, a particular weakness of mine. I decided I'd ring in the New Year with a small scoop. Child-sized. Besides, we had no special plans for the evening, so it seemed a modest and fair thing to have.

Everyone else in line was also waiting to get their proverbial last licks in before the New Year, but all that standing around just made me hungrier and hungrier. I had every intention of getting that child-sized scoop, so I have no idea how I ended up with a two-scoop sundae, but there it was, in my hands, and far be it from me to let it go to waste. The server had been pretty darned chintzy with the whipped cream, but it was a holiday, and I wasn't about to make a scene.

I took my sundae to the car, enjoying a private moment with about 1,500 calories of saturated fat. With every mouthful I thought: This was it. Ice cream and me were kaput, finished, banana splitsville. For me to lose weight, I couldn't have my ice cream and eat it too.

Later on, I was glad I had had my auld lang syne with my ice cream, since my New Year's revelry was pretty much limited to folding laundry, unstopping a toilet, and trying to convince my daughter that all the girls in the second grade did not really hate her.

JANUARY

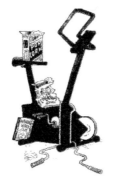

Bound for Glory

January 4

I met a girlfriend for coffee today at a local place legendary
for their pies. She had Boston Crème. I had . . . memories.

January 8

Last night I started Boot Camp! I got off to a rocky start, but
then things improved. I showed up right before 6:00 p.m. at the
park next to the George Page Museum and the La Brea Tar Pits,
which houses dinosaur fossils even older than I am. I spotted
the Major easily. He was the big good-looking brawny guy
wearing Army fatigues and a whistle around his neck. I wanted
to be cool, so I greeted him with, "Hey, Semper Fi, Major!"

"Semper Fi is Marines. This is the Army. We say, 'Hoo-
Yah!'"

"Oh," I said.

"Repeat: Hoo-Yah!"

"Hoo-Yah, Major!"

Then the Major instructed me to get on a scale that he had set down in the parking lot next to his Jeep. I wasn't expecting this, and protested that it was evening, I'd been drinking vats of water all afternoon, and was wearing at least five, maybe even ten pounds of sweat clothes, not to mention shoes, and God knows how much they weighed.

The Major again pointed to the scale. Not wanting to land in the brig for defying an officer who outranked me, especially on the first day, I complied, whining all the while. He took off three pounds for all my stated reasons, but it was still more than my new "Thinner" scale said at home. He was not impressed in the least. Then he did his own fat test, and recorded the information on a chart. This did not entail calipers, as it had at Flab-No-More!, but an odd-looking little handle that I just wrapped my hands around and held out in front of me. Strange how my fingers, my slimmest and perhaps most alluring feature, should provide a fat gauge of my entire body!

After this mortification, for which I had paid pretty big bucks, I asked, "How much weight do you think I should lose, Major?"

He looked me over and said, "Fifteen." Then, reconsidering, he said, "Maybe twenty."

Hoo-Yah, I thought.

I stepped aside as the next recruit took her turn on the scale, and I tried not to grind yet another layer off of my teeth when I heard her squeal that she just couldn't understand how she had *lost* weight over the holidays, what with all the booze she'd been chugging and cheesecake she'd been eating. Some things were just hard to explain.

After proper introductions all around, the Major had us marching, as he directed in a military cadence, "Left, right, left, right, left. Left, right, left, right, left. . ." I was concentrating pretty hard, not wanting to screw up something so simple, but as I was new to the military, I found the atmosphere a little intimidating.

After our march, the Major blew his whistle. "Time to run!

Let's *move!*" he said. We began with a mild jog, and then, when he blew the whistle twice, double-timed it. As we ran, we had to sing. He sang a verse, then we repeated after him. The first few verses went like this:

> "When my granny was ninety-one,
> she did Boot Camp just for fun,
> When my granny was ninety-two,
> she did Boot Camp better than you.
> When my granny was ninety-three,
> she did Boot Camp better than me."

I'm not sure what Granny did for an encore when she turned ninety-four, because I had just collapsed on the side of the track. Meanwhile, the rest of our elite unit sprinted ahead, and I was left behind, no doubt vulnerable to enemy attack. When they came around the track again, I forced my old bones to start running again, and in between my panting breaths, I asked a woman running alongside me, Ziggy, if she had lost any weight since starting Boot Camp. She had done the program several times.

She looked at me as if I were nuts and said, "Hell no! All this exercise makes me hungry!" This concerned me, but I was too out of breath to respond.

Then we had to do as many sit-ups as possible for sixty seconds. During this exercise, the Major called on us, one by one, to reveal what we'd been eating that we should not have been eating. A sorry catalog of edible sins emerged from the mouths of the other recruits: eggnog, éclairs, stuffed pizza, too much beer. I huffed my way through the sit-ups, all the while dreading my turn. When I heard him yell, "Private Gruen!" I figured the sixty seconds were almost up, so I just said, mid-sit-up, "Time's too short for a list that long, Major!"

Fortunately, he did not cite me for insubordination, and I completed the first hour of Boot Camp, completely winded but still raring to go.

January 10

I was not happy today. I weighed in this morning, and given my exemplary behavior in the eating and exercise department lately, I fully expected to see a drop of a pound or two. I didn't think that was too much to ask for. I couldn't believe it when the scale, vicious little machine, said I had gained a pound and a half! I got off the scale. It was early in the morning. My eyes hadn't focused yet. But when I got back on and it said the same vile thing, my mood blackened. I yelled at the kids, listened to bad rock n' roll on the radio, and exhibited other regressive behaviors.

Still fuming, I went out to breakfast and ate and drank everything I wasn't supposed to eat according to the laws of Dr. Charles, Dr. Li, Ingrid, the Major, *Daily Detox Drills,* and *Why Dairy Products Will Kill You!* I had saturated fat in the globs of cheese in my omelet; gluten in my bagel, refined sugar in my crumb donut, and enough caffeine in my three cups of Columbian Supremo coffee to jump start a 747. I avoided complex carbohydrates all day long, because I figured life was already complex enough. If I had been in a better mood, I would have remembered to celebrate the birthdays of George Foreman and Rod ("Do Ya Think I'm Sexy?") Stewart.

I was so frustrated. All that work! All that exercising! My family hadn't seen me in street clothes in two weeks, and I'd GAINED weight? Why did the world have to be so unjust? Later, I met a friend at the market who had the nerve to congratulate me on my weight gain, saying it must mean I was packing on muscle, which as everyone knows weighs more than fat! I almost slapped her.

I thought about the Richard Simmons exercise videos, where at the end, the folks who performed in the video danced forward, one at a time, and were introduced: "Sheila Butagofsky – lost fifty-nine pounds! "Harold Pifvilger – lost 112 pounds!" If I were on the video, it would say "Judy Gruen – gained seventeen pounds!"

Still in a funk, I called my friend Robin, who had lost sixty pounds on Weight Watchers. Surely she would understand. I told her what happened. "Spare me. I ate from midnight to five a.m. since my job is stressing me out so much. Don't sweat it. You'll lose something next week."

Well, I'm no quitter, so in the afternoon, I decided to get back on the wagon. I popped in another Richard Simmons tape. In a perverse way, the guy was growing on me, and besides, I needed some comic relief. "Dancing to the Oldies" was just the right medicine, and seeing Richard doing karaoke to "It's My Party" made the world seem a bit of a sillier, happier place. I sang my own version:

> "It's my weigh-in and I'll cry if I want to,
> cry if I want to, cry-ay-ay if I want to!
> You would cry too if it happened to-oo you-oo!"

I liked the oldies so much and found Richard's kitschy manner so hilarious, I had no trouble getting into the spirit again. After each "oldie" song ended, Richard, choreographer to the corpulent, would shout with joy, clap his hands and run around and hug somebody. I think he was just happy that none of his extra-plus-sized guys and gals dancing around hadn't fallen down and had a stroke during the previous number. I have to hand it to these folks, though. You couldn't get me to perform on a video like that, being that big and wearing those kinds of clothes, unless I was in the Federal Witness Protection Program.

January 11

I have my first battle injury. Running up a hill and through some shrubbery at Boot Camp last night, I sustained a really big scratch along my leg. This is my first war wound, and I already plan to brag about it to my grandchildren. I also hurt just about everyplace from my first two sessions of Boot Camp. My armpits hurt from all the Army-style push-ups, which are feet down, not knees down. Yikes! My thighs are sore from the leg lifts, and nobody better say anything funny because it would really hurt to laugh. These sit-ups have given an unpleasant shock to my stomach muscles, which are being forcibly awakened from their Rip Van Winkle slumber.

However, I see progress already. On only the second night of Boot Camp, I ran longer than twenty-five seconds, and I sure was glad, since the song was even more compelling than the one about Granny's stamina on the running track. As usual, the Major sang a line, and then we had to repeat:

> "We want to live like Airborne Rangers!
> We live lives of sex and danger!
> Airborne rangers! Sex and danger!
> Airborne rangers! Sex and danger!"

Truth to tell, I felt a bit silly singing this song. After all, I'm an old-fashioned Jewish mother of four whose active duty has pretty much been constrained to getting kids to pick up their dirty socks from the floor and forcibly stuffing thirty-pound backpacks into the minivan, and here I was, singing about the exotic lifestyle of America's military heroes and their escapades, both in and out of the barracks! Perhaps this is why I felt a *frisson* of excitement down my spine.

My leg got scratched after we finished running around the track and were busily dashing up a hill where we practice all kinds of daring missions. As a Boot Camp warrior, I was stoic about the injury and continued to train with the rest of the unit. I do hope that in real life, the Army doesn't do so many things backwards, as we do. Otherwise, I would fear for our national safety. For example, the Major has us run up the hill backwards, and down again backwards. We do a "crab crawl" on our hands and feet, also backwards, up that hill. During our crab crawl, someone pointed out a rustling in the tree across the way, and I hoped it wasn't a spy from the enemy's camp. You never know what kind of danger may stalk new Army recruits.

We all enjoyed some comic relief when we were stretching. While all waving our arms around, one gal suddenly shrieked. A piece of wire from her bra had come flying off! Fortunately, nobody was hurt by this underwire friendly fire. Nearing the end of the class, as we were doing yet another set of sit-ups, the Major congratulated us on our form and stamina. He assured us that we must have burned at least 300 calories that evening so far. I asked, "What's that in Danish?"

"Danish?" the Major asked, perplexed. "I don't know any Danish."

Not the language, I thought to myself, the pastry! Would this equate to a half a Danish? A whole Danish? Clearly the Major and I were not on the same wavelength.

When we are all done, our entire unit huddles together, like they do in professional sports games, and performs the sacred ritual of the laying on of hands. Then we yell, "WARRIORS!" After that, we all pick up our water bottles and head home. But last night, as I turned to head toward the car, the Major tapped me on the shoulder and said, "Next time, I want to see your eating log. Write down everything you eat and show it to me, okay?"

"I thought the military had a 'Don't ask, don't tell' policy, Major."

"Not about something as critical to national security as food, Private."

Fearing a court martial for non-compliance, I just yelled, "Hoo-yah, Major."

January 13

I had hoped that the Major would forget about having asked me to write down what I had been eating. Tonight I tried to sneak past him, moving straight to the grass area where we begin our drills.

"Where are you running so fast, missy?" he asked. "Let's see that eating log you promised me."

Reluctantly, I pulled the damning document from my sweater pocket and handed it to him. He looked at it, poker-faced. His review was giving me an anxiety attack, even though in my opinion, I hadn't been that bad. When he finished, he looked at me and said, "You are not going to lose weight by eating two hamburgers and a bun for dinner, even if you didn't put any salad dressing on your salad. You only need to eat what can fit in your fist at each meal, and no more."

"But I was so hungry after our workout. . ."

"See this?" The Major showed me his cupped fist. "That's all the protein you get at a meal. If you get hungry later at night, eat a slice or two of turkey."

Easy for him to say! You could fit a T-bone steak in one of the Major's mammoth paws. I looked at my own fist, which had never before seemed so small. Puny, even, especially if I had to measure my food in it. Was it my fault that the good Lord gave me a hearty appetite?

"And that's another problem with this log," he continued. "You're waiting way too long between meals. Look at your entry from yesterday. You waited almost seven hours after breakfast to eat again, and you made it even worse by topping off breakfast with a cinnamon bun. What were you thinking? You need to eat the right kind of foods every three or four hours or else your body will think it's starving. If it has to worry about where its next meal is coming from, it will slow down your metabolism and will start eating away at your muscle, not your fat."

Slow down my metabolism? A dire threat! I already was convinced that my metabolism was so sluggish that it qualified as a "special needs" bodily system, perhaps even eligible for federal assistance. It needed jump-starting, all right. But was the Major correct about all this? I had just heard a diet doctor on the radio saying that I should keep *longer* intervals between meals to shed pounds, but the Major insisted the opposite was true. Also, I couldn't believe that after more than forty years, my body still didn't trust that I would feed it. Had I ever let it starve before? I did not want to believe the Major when he said that my body was that stupid. I mean, it was smart enough to have made four fully functioning babies, wasn't it? And it was smart enough to produce enough milk for all of them for as long as they wanted, wasn't it? So how could it be dumb and untrusting enough that it would leech away at my muscle if my big crime was waiting six hours between meals?

"Okay, I'll try to do better," I said, crestfallen.

"Remember, every three or four hours you've got to eat a mini-meal, especially protein. Then you just watch that weight fall off!"

That night at dinner, Jeff and the kids wondered why I kept cupping my hand and looking at it sadly before serving myself anything at the table. But I was too tired to explain.

January 15

Haven't had much time to write since I've been busy drinking water. Oceans of water, but the good news is that my initial weight gain of a pound and a half is now gone and I am even down by a half-pound. At this rate, I have to be grateful even for these measly scraps of success. The Major says that each day we should drink half of our body weight in water. I was alarmed until I realized he meant in ounces. But even this command-ment means I must drink rivers full of water, and frankly it's a little hard to get much done when I need to trot off to the kitchen to refill my water bottle many times a day, not to men-tion the resulting bathroom breaks. I'm afraid to even see the water bill this month! And while I'm on the topic of water, I have yet to find a satisfactory answer to the question of why, if our bodies are more than sixty percent water anyway, do we need to drown our insides with even more? And if my body is really sixty percent water, aren't my extra pounds just a bit of water retention?

I also don't understand why the Major and all the other health guides I have listened to or read recently refuse to allow coffee as one of our eight glasses per day. After all, what the heck is coffee but water, brewed in some nice, aromatic little beans? And what about tea? Diet sodas?

When I made the mistake of asking the major about drinking Diet Coke, he said, "If you put a piece of steak in a glass of Coke, it will be gone in two days."

Well, that didn't surprise me. Obviously the dog would get to it.

But he still maintained that if I drank a can of diet soda, which I would do at my own peril, I'd have to drink one and a half times that much more in plain water to make up for its diuretic effects! But drinking water is also a diuretic, if we define that as making us go tinkle really soon after drinking it. Despite my doubts, I am persevering and drinking gallons of water. Supposedly, my bladder will expand its capacity to hold all this water, just as my stomach supposedly will shrink as I become more miserly with the amounts of food I allow in it. But that hasn't happened yet, which reminds me: I have to go now.

January 16

I've been dieting and exercising like a maniac for three weeks now, and so far, Jeff has lost two pounds. Doesn't that just figure? Serves me right for marrying a man who is as indifferent to food as I am to a sale on two-by-fours at Home Depot. Jeff, God bless him, is the kind of man who might not notice if no one ever offered him dessert again for the rest of his life. The only thing he might notice is that if his wife were similarly deprived, she would be stomping around the house in a militant mood, pawing through the freezer in search of a hunk of old birthday cake with freezer burn.

Everyone knows that women can sweat for ten hours a week

on a Stairmaster and live on rice cakes and celery soup and still struggle to lose two pounds, but a man who just eats one burger for dinner instead of two and says the words, "Make it a Bud Light" drops twenty immediately. Another diet book I just read, *Cro-Magnon Menu Magic*, explains why this is so. Apparently, the idea harkens back to prehistoric times, when frequent famines made women, as child-bearers, more important than men in the evolutionary scene. Therefore, we women learned to store our fat efficiently! Thanks, great-great-great-great-great-great-great-great Grandma! I always knew there would never be true equality between the sexes.

January 18

Dieting has reconfirmed a belief that I have held for most of my life, namely, that I particularly do not like the sensation of being hungry. It makes me a little ornery. Once I read an article about Leona Helmsley, that millionaire hotel owner in New York who ended up in a big heap of trouble over some discrepancy between what she thought she owed the government in taxes (she claimed this was about seventy-nine dollars and ninety-five cents), and what Uncle Sam thought she owed (about $42 million). One of old Leona's hotel employees attributed her crack management skills to her eating habits. She said that the woman hardly ate, was always hungry, and more than a tad nasty as a result. Interesting. I never read that in *The Millionaire Next Door* or any other management guide.

But I did just read that government scientists think that living with excruciating hunger — for decades at a time — is actually the ticket to living into Extreme Elderhood. Leave it to the government to come up with a wacky idea like this. But apparently it works. These madcap scientists performed kamikaze calorie-cutting of thirty percent on the diets of such innocent and unsuspecting life forms as yeast, water fleas, and spiders, and found that these same life forms began to live longer, also by as much as thirty percent!

I don't know where all the animal rights activists were while these poor spiders and water fleas were being starved, and I certainly can't imagine just who benefits from a burgeoning population of elderly yeast and wheelchair-bound spiders. But nobody asked me.

When the scientists moved up the low-calorie food chain and found that this draconian diet also helped dogs and monkeys live into decrepitude, they decided to zoom in for the kill with humans. Now, we have thousands of men and women out there who have actually *volunteered* to nibble their way to antiquity. They're part of a grass-roots movement (grass roots is probably all they eat) that survives on fewer calories a day than are in an average large latte and oversized muffin. Only archeologists will finally be able to determine how old these pantaloons were when they finally put that second foot in the grave. One of the male volunteers said he just wants to live to see his great-great-great-grandchildren.

But I doubt that his great-great-great grandchildren will ever see him. I saw this guy's photo in the newspaper, and I've seen POWs hunkier than this man, who subsists on a daily diet of not much more than alfalfa sprouts, a thimbleful of fish and the occasional blueberry. He is six feet tall but weighs only 115 pounds.

Even the government scientists admit that while these wraith-like fellow citizens have fewer colds and flu than the rest of us, food deprivation has its trouble areas. For one thing, just like with Leona Helmsley, chronic hunger makes them snappish. And in men, the complete absence of T-bone steaks also causes another "T" word, namely, testosterone, to plummet, making them lose interest in sex. Despite this, the wife of one of the guys in this program is upset because – I'm not kidding here – all his effort in slicing up raw vegetables for his dinner messes up the kitchen! Hey lady, I have a tip for you: If your husband is six feet tall, weighs less than your vacuum cleaner, and has lost interest in sex, you've got bigger problems than broccoli sprouts on your counter!

I'd much rather live to ninety and have something soft for my great-grandchildren to hug when they see me (and they had better visit, after all I've done for them), than live to 150 and have them wave to me from a distance, an ossified ancestor, for fear that I will turn to dust if they touch me.

January 19 – (down by two pounds!)

I love Boot Camp! Each session gets a little more challenging than the one before, and last night was a blast. I arrived full of energy, since I have finally lost two entire pounds, and am also feeling peppier and more energetic. Tonight we did arduous leg work and weight-lifting before dodging enemy fire, leaping over land mines and performing other feats of military precision. The Major warned that anyone who accidentally exploded a mine (meaning, they tripped over the bar that acted in the place of the real mine) would force the entire unit to do extra push-ups. Now, even though I've improved in many areas at Boot Camp, leaping and vaulting over anything higher than a street curb has never been my forte. So while I successfully dodged the enemy fire through our obstacle course, I was, sadly, the only private in the unit to explode a mine. But my unit has such esprit d'corps, no one complained when we had to get down on the cold wet grass for another series of punishing push-ups, all because of me.

It made me proud to be an American.

January 25

I really asked for it this time. Stupid, stupid, stupid! I'm so frustrated at my body's refusal to let go of more than two pounds, so at Ingrid's urging, I went to visit a holistic physician for advice. (I should have known better than to listen to someone who sends me e-mails with recipes for things like "Barley-Mint Chewies.") And I should have run the other way as soon as I saw how skinny Dr. Tostarella was, since at least I would have gotten some exercise that way. Who could trust anyone wearing a size two skirt to give satisfactory diet advice?

The doctor also trafficked in magnets for necklaces and shoes. I'd heard about these magnets already. Supposedly, they helped you achieve an amazing stress-free existence, hormonal balance, and for all I know, insights into the afterlife. One mother I met at a Little League basketball game practically forced me to wear one of these necklaces, and asked me to host a sales party for her magnetized jewelry. I never did.

I knew I was sunk as soon as I entered Dr. Tostarella's office. She must have gone to the same school as Dr. Li, because the first thing she did was ask me to stick out my tongue slowly, several times. Talk about gauche behavior! I felt really rude but she asked for it, so I stuck my tongue out at her, slowly, as she busily jotted down notes.

After much furrowing of her brow and note-taking, she said, "Not a terrible tongue, but I've seen better." Then she asked me all kinds of off-the-wall questions, such as did I sleep on my left or right side, did I ever dream about unicorns, and did I crave ice shavings. This, apparently, was based on the homeopathic philosophy that only a deep and esoteric knowledge about a person will enable the practitioner to prescribe an appropriate health routine and remedy.

The bad news came fast enough. Based on my "profile," string bean Tostarella (which rhymes with mozzarella, a substance she would eat only after being offered radioactive waste as the alternative) suggested the following diet for me:

First thing in the morning I was to drink a variety of hot teas, especially with ginger, and have fruit so ripe that in another hour it would belong in the compost pile. I could also have, if I was in a jaunty mood, amaranth, which I have never heard of and so don't know whether to buy it in a health food store or a fabric shop. I started writing it all down, but when she said, "And no coffee," my hands began to shake.

I was supposed to lunch on fish, chicken or tofu with a

huge salad that needed to be eaten in a glass bowl, preferably blue. My salads should be tasty tidbits of arugula, spinach, red cabbage, and at least one whole red pepper. I could sprinkle this with raw apple cider vinegar or grapeseed oil if I wished. As she considered further lunch possibilities she looked at me and said, "Try not to have tofu more than three times a week." On this, I gave her my solemn word. Dr. Tostarella was concerned that I was too acidic, and needed to become more "alkaline," as if I'm a battery or something.

Based on this Spartan menu, I was sure I'd be ravenous all day. I didn't want to seem like a total wimp, but I asked what I could eat for an afternoon snack, assuming I hadn't fainted from hunger by this point. She gave me a sideways look, as if this was a very odd question, and replied that I could have as much vegetable juice as I wanted.

I noticed that the more dietary directions she gave me, the more cramped my writing became, as I imagined that finally, as the Major had predicted, my body would have a good reason to feel I was starving it to death. Dinner would be the most exciting meal of the day, starring cooked kale and red onions, shitake mushrooms, green and orange vegetables, and root vegetables, such as rutabaga. Dr. Tostarella advised that I have three pots on the burners each night, so as to cook each vegetable combination appropriately. I could also have a baked potato, millet or brown rice with hummus.

I said, "What about a bedtime snack? I usually like something sweet at night. Can I at least have a fruit?"

Dr. Tostarella shot me a look that would have seared tofu. She shrugged her shoulders, as if to insinuate that only a glutton would fail to find this menu immensely satisfying.

"Never eat fruit after ten o'clock in the morning. Fruit after protein ferments in the system, and besides, your digestive system shuts down after eight p.m. If you really want something late at night, have a few sprouted almonds," she said, rising from her chair and indicating our session was over. "And remember the most important rules: no refined sugar, no white flour, no coffee, no dairy, no red meat. Almost every disease process in the human body comes from dead animal flesh."

There was something about Dr. Tostarella's tone that set my potatoes steaming. How the hell did she know what time my digestive system shut down for the night? Maybe my digestive system was really nocturnal by nature, like our hamsters. Maybe my digestive system was a highly motivated self-starter, and didn't have that kind of annoying, bureaucratic, clock-watching attitude so pathetically common among internal organs nowadays. Worse, who did this diaphanous doctor think she was, sneering at my sugar addiction? Trying to take away my coffee, my sugar, my cheese, even my burgers! How, for example, did she expect me to commemorate in a fitting manner the late General Douglas MacArthur's birthday, and the anniversary of the television premiere of "The Dukes of Hazard," both of which were today?

"Look doc," I said, trying to stay calm even though I hadn't had any chocolate in about four hours, "coffee will never, ever be on the negotiating table. And the only way anyone will take away my chocolate will be to pry it from my cold, dead fingers. *Capish*?"

"It's your life," she said, shaking her head in disgust. "Just remember my motto: 'Fermentation Happens.'"

I don't know why, but I left Dr. Tostarella's office determined to try her nutball diet.

January 30

Ingrid keeps e-mailing me, wanting to know about my progress with the reunion and with my weight loss program. What a nag! I'm beginning to think we ought to just throw a Virtual Reunion online. That would save me an awful lot of trouble.

Obviously I haven't had the nerve to suggest this to Ingrid, and besides, I feel I've thrown down the gauntlet. While my weight loss is unimpressive so far, I feel great. The kids have all been sick, but, unlike previous winters, I haven't caught anything from them! There must be something to eating all these collard greens after all.

Ingrid and I have set June 30 as the date for the reunion, which means I have exactly 158 days to lose another thirteen pounds.

FEBRUARY

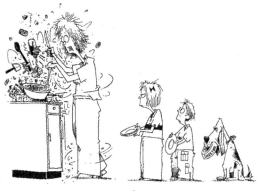

Mission: Improbable

February 2

I am rather put out that this whole process is taking so long. So, still searching for the Holy Grail of nutritional advice, I took some more books out from the library. I was intrigued by one called *Eat Your Blood Type or Else!* which featured heavy black and red type on the cover and an exclamation point in the title that scared me. The author of the book, a Dr. Pocket, insisted that my blood type explained my predicted longevity, vitality, emotional strength, and probably, my preference for mid-19th century British authors. I zoomed straight toward the section of the book on my blood type, "O." I was riveted by Dr. Pocket's explanation that monarchies, tribes, even entire civilizations have been built on nothing more substantial than blood ties, and even more fascinated to learn that somehow, all this history led to the conclusion that I should not eat oat fiber or buffalo. After all, as a Type O, I was part of the oldest living blood type, descendents of determined Cro Magnon carnivore ancestors who had zero tolerance for competitors for the meat available on the savannah. I imagined my knuckle-dragging ancestors walking around, wielding clubs and wearing team t-shirts emblazoned with the words "No Fear." In fact, this intense competition for meat, even to the death, sounded vaguely familiar. In fact, it sounded like hamburger night at my house.

While in a way I was gratified to learn that my blood type had played such a distinguished role in the evolutionary chain, I began to tune out when Dr. Pocket explained more about the basis for his theory. This included something about forced migrations from Africa into Europe and Asia and my ancestors' first harsh realization that they would have to start eating berries, nuts, grubs, and, in a pinch, frozen yogurt from the local mini-mart.

Eat Your Blood Type or Else! also claimed that Type Os still prefer foods that we could hunt and kill ourselves, such as bison. Frankly, hunting for a choice cut of shoulder roast at the butcher counter on a busy day at my local market does bear some similarities to what my ancestors had to endure. In fact, there have been times when I wished I had a club myself, especially when I finally got out of the store and saw someone with an SUV the size of Houston blocking my car. Due to an unfortunate twist of gastrointestinal fate, Dr. Pocket claimed that some foods contained particular types of protein lectins that have become, over time, my mortal enemies! Eating these bad foods would cause no end of trouble for me, including bloating, toxins polluting my innards, throwing off my hormonal balance, and forgetting to take the car for an oil change.

Somehow, even though 25,000 years have passed, Dr. Pocket believed that we Type Os are still "not used to" dairy products – after all, you don't have to chase down and kill a bowl of yogurt! The list of banned foods for Type Os was a long and sorry one, and included bagels, muffins, corn, kidney beans, nearly all dairy products, strawberries, red potatoes, goose, barracuda and octopus. Admittedly, I can get along fine without the octopus and barracuda, but lentils? Supposedly, lentils made me too "alkaline," but Dr. Tostarella said I needed to become *more* alkaline!

I get mighty suspicious when supposed experts tell us that foods filled with vitamins, minerals and fiber are not good for us. Recently, I asked my hairdresser, Lori, what was the worst diet she had ever tried. She answered in a snap, "Dr. Atkins, for sure! How can you trust a guy who tells you that bacon is fine but a tomato is bad?"

I had to agree with her. Dr. Pocket and Dr. Tostarella could duke it out if they liked over the issue of lentils and my ideal alkaline quotient, but in the meantime, I plan to eat lentils, and strawberries, with impunity. Unfortunately, the only thing these two agreed on was that I should cut coffee from my diet – dreamers, both of them.

February 3

Amazingly, I survived nearly an entire week on a modified version of Dr. Tostarella's program. It wasn't always easy. Last night, Jeff and I went out to dinner to one of our favorite places, which serves fabulous Persian food. Searching for a menu selection that Dr. Tostarella would approve of was like mining for gold in the Sudan.

"What? No brown rice?" I said, never having noticed before the omission of this choice food item. Since it was past one o'clock in the afternoon, I had to rule out chicken, fish, and beef. Noodles and white rice were out of the question, as were most of the other 169 tantalizing offerings on the menu.

This was supposedly a chance for Jeff and me to relax and enjoy one another's company, but ordering my dinner became stressful for both of us. Long after he had finished his first beer, I was still lost in concentration behind the oversized menu.

"The baby-sitter needs to be home by nine-thirty," Jeff reminded me, a tad testily.

Soon, the waiter also marched over to show us the "no loitering" clause written in small print at the bottom of the menu, which was when I realized that the organic ink used to print said clause was one of the only allowable things on my diet. By the time I ordered a plate of mixed stir-fried vegetables, a side order of hummus, and, in a major capitulation, white rice, I was so hungry I thought I would faint.

Lucky for me, I really do enjoy lots of vegetables and brown rice, so overall, I actually did pretty well on Dr. Tostarella's regimen for the first few days. I took particular pleasure in my morning coffee, just knowing that she would disapprove. But by midweek, my enthusiasm flagged. I wondered why I had heartburn all afternoon, until I realized the culprit had to have been all those raw red peppers and greens I was eating every day at lunch. Frankly, I wasn't willing to pay that high a price for optimal health. By late in the week, I threw caution to the wind and did the unthinkable: I ate an apple at four o'clock in the afternoon. I was also bothered by the fact that this routine directly contradicted the Major's exhortations to eat every three hours, especially protein. He was even big on tossing back a few turkey slices before bed, an idea that probably would have put Dr. Tostrarella into cardiac arrest.

And I had other problems with this routine. First, I had to cook separate dinners for the kids and for me, which was more work than I had time for each afternoon. And, I tried feeding Jeff the same things I ate, not because the man carries even a single excess pound, but just in the interest of his overall health. However, he discovered that an all-vegetable dinner still left a gaping hole in his appetite, and the poor man was hungry for the rest of the evening. Jeff is not the kind of guy who snacks, so when I saw him looking forlornly in the refrigerator at ten p.m., I knew something had to give. Finally, there was only so much kale I could eat in a week.

For all these reasons, I decided to transfer my eating allegiance to the Major, and began making further modifications to my diet based on my most convincing evidence so far. This doesn't count the apple fritter I had yesterday, which was strictly for mental health. What else could I do? I had had one of those days. The kitchen sink backed up again, not a week after paying for all new plumbing underneath. The kids, whose idea of a term of endearment for one another is "Hey, slog brain!" were fighting over computer time, who ate the last ice cream bar, whose turn it was to set the table, and whose bad breath was making them ill. My brand new chenille sweater snagged on a nail sticking out of a door and began to unravel faster than my nerves.

As an aside, it has always seemed to me that aggravation endured by mothers in the line of duty should burn calories and lead to weight loss. The more kids a woman has, the more aggravation she has, and therefore the thinner she has a right to be. Mothers of more than three kids, or even a single teenager, would be invisible. But it doesn't work this way. One of the nutrition books I read recently, and also rejected, was called, *Sniffing Your Way Svelte.* This guy's premise is that what most overweight people really crave is not food, but food aromas! He advises buying this funny inhaler that emits pleasant food aromas that somehow will tell our bodies that we are quite satiated, thank you, and we will eat less and lose weight.

Anyway, I am eating fruit in the morning, but with fat-free cottage cheese, which is okay by me. I gave up on all those fresh bitter salads, since it is February and according to my calendar it is soup season. I'm eating healthfully, have cut out most bread, and am still eating mustard greens and millet — within reason.

February 4 (down four pounds!)

Today I successfully faced one of the greatest character tests of my entire life. I had to get up at five-thirty a.m. to get to Boot Camp by six o'clock. We were having final evaluations and graduation, and since I couldn't make the evening class that I usually attend, I had no choice but to go at this beastly hour.

I have never been a morning person. Come to think of it, I'm not much of a night person, either, but I have a pretty good stretch of alertness between nine-thirty a.m., after breakfast, and about four p.m. It's usually all downhill from there. But after four weeks of Boot Camp with the Major, there's no way would

I miss my moment of glory! I even harbored a fantasy the Major would make me a lieutenant in recognition of my bravery on the front lines.

I bounded out of bed at the stroke of five-thirty, quickly getting into my workout clothes, and drove away. I had no idea it was still dark outside at this hour, which made me feel even more heroic than I already felt. I was the first to arrive at Boot Camp, and sat shivering in the car. It was cold! No more than forty-five degrees, tops. When the rest of the recruits arrived, everyone had been smart enough to bring gloves. Everyone, that is, except me.

Just as he had the first day of Boot Camp, the Major had his scale and fat calculator ready. Oh, the suspense of it all! What would I have to show for all my hard work? All those push-ups on the cold, wet grass, at an uphill incline? All those bicep and tricep curls? Running forwards and backwards on the hill? Memorizing all those Army cadences? By now, I could sing my way all the way from Fort Ord to Fort Bragg. My heart raced as I stepped on the scale, but at least I wasn't yammering and griping as I had during the first weigh-in. I held my breath in anticipation.

Hallelujah! On the Major's scale, I lost *four* pounds since the Boot Camp had begun and had even gained one pound of muscle! I was so happy, not to mention freezing cold, that I starting running around the track. When I returned from my victory lap, a few other recruits sauntered over to introduce themselves. Since I was a member of the evening class, they didn't know me, but they were a friendly bunch. One guy strode over and extended his hand.

"Hi, I'm Larry, eighteen percent body fat," he said.

"Hi, I'm Judy," I said, before suffering a sudden and unexplainable coughing fit, rendering anything else I said inaudible. Only a man would introduce himself that way.

Happily, I performed better on every exercise than I had four weeks earlier. I did more sit-ups, more push-ups, more flutter kicks, and even more squat-thrusters. (Squat-thrusters are embarrassing to pronounce and even more embarrassing to do.) In fact, I did more everything than I had at the beginning, and with better form. I even trimmed about fifteen seconds off our running course, even if I was still the last one back. But so what? I was exercising at six in the morning, and I would have felt just about invincible if not for the frostbite developing on my toes. I comforted myself that shivering burns calories.

At the end of our evaluations, we stood in formation and waited for the Major to call us by name and present us with a certificate and Boot Camp Warrior t-shirt. When he called, "Recruit Gruen! In recognition of your hard work, dedication to the team, and never once uttering the words 'Dove Bars' or 'Little Debs', I hereby award you this certificate." I stepped forward, had a photo-op with the Major, and got back in line, almost insufferably delighted with myself. The Major announced that we were all on furlough for the entire weekend.

I was so proud! When I came home, I annoyed the children by marching into the house and loudly singing a military song that extolled the virtues of blowing up enemies in a foreign land. It really was a catchy tune, and I had sung several verses before realizing this might not be the most appropriate morning wake-up song for four impressionable children.

When my teenage son complained about my good humor, a trait that makes teens violently ill, I got in his face and snarled, "Watch it, mister. I'm a Boot Camp warrior, and if you ever talk to me like that again, you'll do twenty push-ups before you see breakfast." Boy did that shut him up!

I am so ashamed that in my youth I made fun of the military.

February 5

I think I went a little overboard with the furlough business. At first, I was going to allow myself only one cinnamon bun. Just one. I figured it would be nice if the whole family could sit around and enjoy them together on Sunday morning. The problem was, when I tucked into the first one on Friday after coming home from the market, I became heady with excitement. It had been such a long time since I'd had one of these! At least, it *seemed* to be a long time.

On Sunday morning, still sound asleep, I was awakened by a familiar racket in the kitchen. This usually indicates that the Toasty-Smacks cereal is nearly gone, and the kids are fighting over the last morsels. But this exchange grew more heated than usual, so I had to lug myself out of bed to investigate. Much to my horror, my eldest was waving the now-empty box that had contained the cinnamon buns.

"Who ate them all? I didn't get any!" he shouted.

"Not me! I only ate one! I was allowed one!" chimed another, defending his name.

One by one, they declaimed responsibility for strafing the sweets. I knew where this was going, and it wouldn't be pretty. Then, as if sharing a communal revelation, eight accusing eyes turned to me. I was wearing an old bathrobe and a guilty expression. It was over.

"Okay, you caught me. I ate three of them. Sorry! Next time I won't touch them," I confessed. It was really much too early in the morning for this type of confession.

"I thought you were on a diet," one child asked, a child who would have the audacity to ask me to cook his dinner that night and give him a raise in his allowance.

"Yes, well. . ."

"Leave Mom alone. She's had a hard week," said Jeff, coming to my rescue, though I didn't deserve it. "Everyone around here eats too much sugar as it is."

I skedaddled out of the room and into workout clothes, preparing to do penance.

February 8

Despite my having overdone the furlough bit, I am back on track now. I am pursuing a goal that proves once again the triumph of hope over experience. In fact, if I eat any more turnip greens this week I will probably start talking like Butterfly McQueen in "Gone With the Wind." If I chew any more raw carrots the whites of my eyes will turn orange. And, it has been thirty-seven days since I have eaten any real ice cream — an unheard-of achievement for me. I think the city should name a street after me or something. This whole enterprise had better be worth it.

February 10

With Boot Camp over, I had to keep the momentum going. Because the truth is, eating dark leafy vegetables, even in alarming volume, is not likely in and of itself to lead to my gaining a stunning physique. Despite my aversion to counting calories and quantifying my food portions, I did something else radical and joined Weight Watchers. Fortunately, Weight Watchers has evolved from the old days when you had to carry around these little packets of two-calorie salad dressing that smelled like rancid vinegar and tasted worse. These days, you have to carry around a little calculator that figures out the "points" in the food you eat. Sophisticated Weight Watchers, however, go way beyond that. They are part of a loyal Weight Watchers *gemeinschaft*, and are often seen wearing their little Weight Watchers pedometers, which tell them how far they are walking, and how many calories they are burning during their daily existence, including when they tie their shoes or scratch their noses. They carry around their Weight Watchers water vats and are never seen without their Weight Watchers diaries in which they dutifully record every morsel of food or drink that passes their lips. When they are hungry, they have an arsenal of Weight Watchers "nutritional snack bars," the better to ward off a sudden Big Mac attack. All these accessories can be carried around handsomely in a leatherette Weight Watchers pouch, so as to better organize the entire Weight Watchers lifestyle.

Depending on your weight, you are allowed a certain range of points per day on this program. You don't have to count calories or weigh food, which is a huge relief and at the same time, surely a disappointment to all those manufacturers of little kitchen scales. The good news is that I am in the lowest weight category for inclusion in the program. The bad news: I get the fewest points per day!

I was amazed to see hordes of people jamming the hallway trying to get into the Weight Watchers meeting. You'd think we were waiting for some hotly anticipated Hollywood movie premiere, where we might even see Tom Cruise and his really white teeth. Instead, we were lined up, waiting to fork over more than the price of a movie ticket for the entertainment of having a thin stranger put us on a scale and write the measurement down on a chart for posterity. There is some privacy, as we are weighed in a little booth that is kind of like a voting booth, only here we don't have the option of selecting a "write-in" candidate for our weight. There are limits to democracy in Weight Watchers.

Predictably, ninety percent of those in line were women, but many of them were already slim. I felt like asking them, "Hey! What are *you* doing here?" But I quickly realized that they probably only got that way from the program and came for moral support. While I filled out my application to join, I saw veteran members hunting down their membership cards in boxes on a table. I realized that a sneaky person could surreptitiously peek at other people's cards and see how much they weighed. Could anybody really stoop that low? I looked around at the group. They seemed to have honest faces, but you never can tell.

After we weigh in, our group leader, a formerly adipose person, gives a pep talk. Carmen inspires hope in the hippy by saying things like, "Remember, if you are really hungry, a banana is only two points!" Yet she doesn't shy away from chastising either. "Look, friends, if you insist on going out to dinner four times a week and tucking into an eighteen-point bowl of pasta carbonara, don't come crying to me if you gain weight that week!" Carmen calls them like she sees them: "Nothing tastes as good as thin feels," she says.

More shocking than the sheer numbers at the meeting, though, was the discovery that I knew about every other person in the room! I saw teachers from the kids' school, neighbors, even a woman in the book club I used to belong to. I felt as if I had joined some secret society where everyone spoke in code. After my weigh-in, I overheard this conversation:

"Yesterday I ate a five at two and then I had a ten at seven, but it's okay because I had banked four points from last week and knew I would eat them yesterday."

"Lucky you! I ate more than thirty points on Saturday so only had fifteen yesterday, so I tried to eat around a four every four hours."

The sick thing was, I followed what they were saying! The idea of banking points was lost on me; I knew that my account would probably always be overdrawn. I did consider taking out stock in the company, though. Most people weren't only paying to weigh in at ten bucks a pop; they were eagerly surrendering their credit cards to pay for all manner of Weight Watcher vendibles: electronic food point calculating devices, online diet support, cookbooks, shake mixes, and magazines. But their biggest seller seemed to be their snack bars, which are made of really scary-sounding things. My chocolate mint bar, for example, includes something called "fructooligosaccharides," which sounds like a cereal from outer space, and "alpha-tocopherol acetate," which never needs ironing. Jammed with these alien-sounding compounds, I doubt whether these bars qualify, strictly speaking, as food. But who cares? These bars only have two points each, so people buy them by the truckload. Even I, who loathe ersatz desserts, sprang for two varieties of chocolate- flavored bars. While waiting in line to pay, a lady behind me tapped me on the shoulder. She was teetering under the weight of about three-dozen boxes of oatmeal raisin while trying to convince me that her flavor was a lot less gummy tasting than the chocolate flavors I had chosen. But she was barking up the wrong tree. My tastes may not be very adventurous, but my motto is if it ain't broke, don't fix it.

The highlight of Carmen's presentation was the awarding of a bookmark, yes, a bookmark, to a guy named Frank who achieved a ten-pound weight loss milestone. We all applauded wildly, as if we were guests in the audience of "Oprah."

I left the meeting with my stack of literature, slide rule, diet diary, and two boxes of two-point snack bars. But I was not happy that they recorded my weight as three pounds heavier than what the Major and I each recorded on our respective scales. I mean, I had lost weight, hadn't I? According to the Major and me, I had lost four pounds, but according to Weight Watchers, I had only lost one. Something was fishy here. For a fleeting moment, I wondered if they padded their scales, to make us think we were fatter than we were. Well, I'll give it a try, though I do think it's rather obsessive-compulsive to have to write down everything you eat.

February 11

My family is in open mutiny against me. Ingrates, all! The insurrection began last night at the dinner table, where most family dramas play out.

"Brown rice and vegetables *again?*" My adolescent asked this question accusingly. As he sees it, it's his job not to like anything.

"What about it? Chinese people eat this type of food every day, and they have almost no heart disease," I said. "Don't you want me to cook healthfully for you?"

That might have qualified for the most stupid rhetorical question ever asked in the history of stupid rhetorical questions. Children would eat their socks if only they were dipped in chocolate and stuck in the freezer for an hour.

"All this healthy food is making us sick. And, if you haven't noticed, Mom, we're not Chinese! We like Chinese food with MSG, from restaurants, but not this!"

"Yeah!"

"Yeah!" They were working up a lather over this, but at least they were united in a cause, instead of fighting as usual.

"But look, you have so much to choose from on the table right now: miso soup, hummus, fish, even potatoes! This is an extremely healthy meal, and you ought to be grateful," I said, wondering why I was on the defensive for trying to take better nutritional care of them. "Don't you realize there are starving children in Africa? They wouldn't complain about a dinner like this! *They* would be grateful!"

"Why are you concerned about strange children starving in Africa when you have your own children starving right here in the kitchen?" my daughter cried.

"Yeah! Besides, we'd be happy to wrap it up and send it to them. If you're that concerned about their welfare, we can even overnight it to them," piled on a sibling. Why did all four of my kids have to be wise guys? Naturally, Jeff was not home yet to bail me out.

"We *were* healthy! We *were* strong! Now we're weak, since *you* haven't bought any ice cream in ten billion bazillion years!" exclaimed my daughter, who boasts that she never exaggerates.

"That's not true!" I said. "I bought two cartons of choco-late-flavored 'Soy Good!' frozen dessert product. No one touched it."

"I tasted it, and it made me throw up!" insisted the adolescent, who was suddenly distracted by the sensation that his feet had just grown another full shoe size.

"Why can't we have real ice cream? Why did you give it to us before if it's so bad?"

"It's not that it's so bad, it's just that. . . it's better if it's not in the house, that's all," I stammered, feeling pathetic.

"Just because *you* needed to lose weight, why are you taking it out on us? What did *we* do?" another son pined. They continued their assault by reminding me that this was Thursday, and Thursday always used to be hot dog night.

"We want hot dogs!"

"Hot dogs! Hot dogs!"

"We'll even clean up the kitchen afterwards!"

It all became too much. I promised to break open a package of hot dogs if they each ate at least two spoonfuls of vegetables and a serving of brown rice. Three of the four had no problem with this, but one son, who refuses to recognize the existence of vegetables, found it tough going. I stood my ground and refused to cook the hot dogs until the vegetables were consumed. When his three siblings threatened a physical attack unless he complied, the vegetable-hater forced the spoonfuls down his gullet.

Eating the hot dogs improved their state of mind, if not their bodies, but that was enough for me. I even promised them ice cream the next day. Trying to look at the bright side, I realized that with all these leftovers, I wouldn't have to cook anything else for myself for several days.

February 13

It's very hard to go to the grocery store so close to Valentine's Day. Today, I saw some spectacle or other of Whitman samplers or Reese's miniature peanut butter cups on almost every aisle. I reminded myself that today was Ash Wednesday and the beginning of Lent, and indulgences of this kind were inappropriate. Then I remembered that I was Jewish and that these prohibitions did not apply to me, but I would try to keep them regardless, in the spirit of achieving my goal.

I tried to push away from my mind the fact that today was both Stockard Channing's and Jerry Springer's birthdays, days that before I began my health regimen I might have celebrated with an apple fritter. This was out of the question now, but I couldn't help but imagine — even though it was just a hunch — that Jerry Springer liked nougats and that Stockard (what an unfortunate name for a woman!) preferred hazelnuts. I was doing okay until I got close to the paper goods area, where I was gob smacked by a dazzling display that was a veritable shrine to the chocolate industry. Red shiny paper gleamed at me from rows of heart-shaped boxes of all sizes, some with lace borders, others with teddy bears: Fanny Farmer chewy pecan dixies, Hershey's kisses and caramel clusters, Dove Truffle hearts (both milk and dark chocolate), and Nestles' turtles, wrapped in a rose ribbon. My pace slackened, and I told myself to keep moving, but I froze in position in front of a box of Mrs. Fields' Decadent Chocolates. I picked up the chocolates and held them close, and then experienced a close encounter of the olfactory kind. I smelled it, testing the theory of that diet doc who claimed that all we really wanted was a good close sniff of a delectable food delight. He was wrong. I looked around to make sure no one was looking, and then I whispered to the box, "One day, you and me, alone at a candle-lit table. Maybe next year." I turned the box over in my hands, hating to pass it up, especially since it was a "key buy" and two bucks off regular price.

But then my new Weight Watchers training kicked in. I realized that a three-piece serving had 220 calories and three Weight Watchers points, but the entire box (a far more plausible calculation) contained an artery-stopping 1,980 calories! I pulled out my Weight Watchers points calculator and found it didn't go that high. It probably packed as many points as I was allotted for a whole week! I compared this with a smaller box of Reese's peanut butter heart-shaped chocolates, which had only 760 calories and forty-four grams of fat for the box. These stopped me cold. But then tears came to my eyes when I saw a Russell Stover assortment with a picture of Elvis Presley on the cover. This box promised to play "Love Me Tender" when opened – truly romantic! I forced myself to replace all the boxes of chocolates, as the store's sound system began broadcasting "I'm Lost Without Your Love."

Even the checkout line held dangers. Not only did I have to go to the bathroom (again), but also a mini-freezer plunked down between two check stands and choked with Häagen-Dazs bars was staring me down. I had to take my mind off things caloric and diuretic and instead turned my attention to the cover of a tabloid newspaper, where I was forced to consider the unsettling possibility that Prince William really was the love child of Diana and a space alien.

February 15

Every single heart-shaped box of Valentine's Day candy at the supermarket is now seventy-five percent off! How could they do this to me? This *must* qualify as a "hostile shopping environment" for dieters. Perhaps government intervention is called for. I did not allow myself to linger over the lonely display, especially since I quickly deduced the following: On sale, I could buy nearly every species of chocolates for just pennies a taste, but losing weight was costly, too. Between what I'd spent so far on Boot Camp, exercise videos, new hand weights, workout clothes, and Weight Watchers meetings, it had cost me nearly a hundred bucks a pound for every pound I've dropped so far! I couldn't afford to keep losing weight at these prices, so I refused to buy Valentines chocolates.

Besides, I don't want to undermine my own extremely meager success so far. My friend Denise told me the other day that my face looks thinner than it had the last time she had seen me. At first, I thought she meant I just looked haggard from chocolate deprivation and slogging around the house hoisting my exploding inventory of hand weights and workout body bars. But then other people started making similar comments, so I just may cancel my order for that "Flab-Free Faceaerobics" video. Maybe I don't even need it anymore!

February 17 (133 days before Coop reunion)

Good news! At my Weight Watchers weigh-in this morning, I lost two and a half pounds! I was so excited, I told a total stranger sitting next to me about my grand success. She looked bored and said, "Yeah, I lost four pounds after my first week." Get that woman a ticket to a Dale Carnegie seminar! Doesn't anyone have any class anymore? It's a good thing I had this victory, since this evening we had another family birthday celebration, and I was faced with the usual fatty deli platter, mayonnaise-choked salads and cake. This time I came prepared by bringing a tray of steamed broccoli, cauliflower and carrots. I also brought a bowl of fresh fruit to distract myself from the inevitable birthday cake.

On Weight Watchers, I can eat as many of the vegetables as I want, since most of them have zero points. I sometimes call these foods "pointless," because you can eat them all day long and still feel hungry. At tonight's party, I just about wore out my poor jawbone chomping on my jicama and snow peas to avoid piling more meat on my plate. I passed on the potato salad, kept pawing through the vegetables, and ate a half a turkey sandwich. By the time dessert came along, though, things got sticky. Relatives kept passing me a hunk of cake, seeming not to notice that I kept saying, "No thank you."

"What's the harm? It's a *birthday*!" a cousin said.

"Yes, I know, but I'm happy with the fruit," I said. I felt tension in the air. I wasn't trying to make anyone feel guilty, but I also didn't need my family trying to shove four hundred and fifty calories worth of cake in front of my face every two minutes, either.

I stayed strong, and eventually they got the message.

February 18

Today I got a call from a guy named Mickey, who asked me why I never returned to "Bodies by Barbarella," a gym near my house where I had received a two-week pass but had only gone two times. When Mickey asked what the problem was, I was blunt.

"Look," I said, "Your brochure says that no experience is necessary, but when I went to Barbarella's step class, I thought I had stumbled into a rehearsal for the Alvin Ailey Dance Troupe. The choreography was great for a Broadway show, but I couldn't keep up. And another thing: I'm not a big fan of techno-rap, especially when it is blasted so loudly that it can cause deafness."

I also complained to Mickey that when I tried to escape the window-rattling volume of the step class, the only place left for me to hide was next to the air conditioner vent, where I caught cold. Even though my first day was such a disaster, I gave the place another chance the next day for a spinning class, only to discover that the class was so popular that people had reserved their bikes with a small deposit months in advance. To add insult to injury, even though I couldn't get into the class, I still had to pay for parking. I felt utterly persecuted by both the fitness and parking industries.

Mickey apologized for my ghastly experiences, and offered to extend my free pass for another week, but I had had enough. Instead, I've been taking fast walks in the neighborhood, making sure to go up hills, and doing some exercise tapes at home. This suits me just fine. At home, I don't have to pay for parking or watch a parade of beautiful people and wonder which components of their too-perfect bodies have been surgically enhanced. At Bodies by Barbarella, I must have seen at least $100,000 worth of tummy tucks, buttock enhancements other marvels of cosmetic surgery in a single room.

I'm glad I pre-screened several exercise videos from the library first before buying any more, since I cannot take most of the instructors without an injection of insulin. I don't know what they drink in the morning, but most of them are just too perky for my taste. You had better like their personalities, too, since they yammer at you for the entire hour. And other than

Richard Simmons, very few instructors employ any pudgy performers. Those who do will have only the Token Plump Person, exerting herself and sweating profusely next to all the Hollywood-thin models. And those fake sets, so stylized and glammed up, can also be a bit much. For one aerobics interval, they're in a Hawaiian garden; the next, they've moved to the beach and changed their color-coordinated costumes, too. Really, now.

So far, my favorite instructor is Karen Voigt, who has tapes to bring out the muscle tone in everything from your fingernails to the soles of your feet. And I can listen to her for a whole tape, since she never acts like a sultry seductress or a cheerleader whose team has just scored a touchdown. She even tells me I'm doing a great job, even if I've stopped for a few moments to throw in a load of laundry. And when her choreography gets a little tricky, I can always press the "rewind" button and do it again.

February 19

Today I heard an advertisement on the radio for a new skin patch that leeches the fat from you. It's called "Skim-Skin" or "Slim-Skin" or something like that. I think the same guy does every single weight-loss commercial I hear on the radio; he has that oily kind of voice. He speaks in a breathless tone, as if he had just fallen off an elliptical bicycle. "Imagine! Eat whatever you want, maintain your usual couch-potato habits and still lose weight! It's amazing but true!" Honestly! This country has more than its share of bamboozlers and charlatans.

February 20 (down five pounds)

Our friends Lawrence and Edie threw a party last night to celebrate their tenth wedding anniversary and laid out a magnificent Viennese table for the occasion. When we arrived, I spotted my girlfriends huddled in a corner next to the elegant spread, so I couldn't very well avoid close contact with the gorgeous desserts. None of my friends were eating anything, probably because Tanya was there, standing like a silent sentry. It would take a lot of gumption to eat white sugar in front of her. I tried to feign interest in their conversation, but my attention was riveted on an enormous chocolate trifle, made in a deep glass bowl, with several repeating layers of chocolate cake and mysterious gooey chocolate formations. The icing on the cake, as it were, included a variety of butterscotch chips, sprinkles, and chocolate shavings. I think it may have qualified as the eighth wonder of the world. It was one of the most beautiful things I had ever seen.

I had to have some.

"Excuse me, girls," I said, slipping away from their circle and over to the table. I pushed away the image of my Weight Watchers diary in my purse, whose pages I hadn't filled for several days. I spooned some of the trifle up onto a plate, and boldly returned to my circle of friends, who were dishing up low-calorie but high-interest gossip about people near and dear to us. I didn't care what Tanya or anybody else thought.

"Yes, Jake is moving to Chicago for that new job in May, and it looks like he'll be marrying Louise after all," said Mona. This was big news, as Jake and Louise had been dating for thirteen years.

"Really? It's about time!" enthused Kate.

"Absolutely. She better hold him to it this time," added Tanya, sipping a Perrier. "Isn't that great news, Judy?"

"Oh my God, there's peanut butter in here," I said, in a trifle-induced reverie. I had no idea what they were talking about.

"And another thing," continued Mona, "Bill's finally been promised that promotion, so I'm going to be able to remodel the kitchen after all!"

"You go, girl!" Tanya said.

"Get the black granite countertop," Kate added. "You know how much you've always wanted it."

"Mint! There are crushed mint cookies in here! Oh my God," I mumbled, in a swoon.

"Poor girl," Mona said to Tanya and Kate, shaking her head sadly. "She needs to get out more."

"She seems kind of delirious to me," Kate said. "Is she on any funny diet pills? You know they haven't done a lot of conclusive studies on the long-term effects of these things."

While my friends were diagnosing my condition, a rude rapscallion of a man came over to me and pointed to my plate. "Do you have any idea how many calories are in there?" he asked.

"What's it to you, pal?" I parried, protectively holding my plate close to my chest, hoping I wouldn't smear chocolate on my blouse.

"Look, I know how hard you've been working on this. Why blow it on a silly dessert? You don't have to eat the whole thing. I'll share with you," offered my husband, the erstwhile rapscallion. He really thought he was being helpful.

"This is MINE," I said. "Every single calorie. Every single point. Every gram of saturated fat. Every granule of sugar. Now back away slowly and you won't get hurt."

I don't know why men have such a poor sense of timing.

On the way home, I tried but failed to feel guilty. Mostly, I felt immense satisfaction in having eaten something so sensually amazing. I was trying to remember the reason why Lawrence and Edie had thrown the party, since I know there was a reason, but all I could think about was the fact that there was still a lot of trifle left in the bowl at the end of the evening.

February 21

I have to confess that I have decided to can all those little jerky, nervous body movements I've been doing lately. I started it a while ago, after reading a magazine article that explained that one reason Type A personalities tend to be thinner than everyone else is because they're always fidgeting, bouncing their knees incessantly, as if they were attached to a spring, shrugging their shoulders and otherwise exerting themselves with no apparent purpose. A little compulsive, I realized, but hey, it burned calories, didn't it? Why, researchers discovered that some really manic Type As might tear through 300 calories a day just being neurotic!

Well, I thought, two can play this game. So, I started aping these weird mannerisms, just like I'd been doing it my whole life: tossing and turning at night, tapping my foot nervously, and craning my neck around, as if I were expecting to be attacked from behind. At the doctor's office, I stood in the waiting room instead of sitting, taking the opportunity to do some bicep curls with a decorative glass bowl filled with marbles. No one said anything at first, and I was sure I was furthering my quest for a smaller body from all this mindless mobility. But then the other day, my neighbor Lisa saw me at the market and spied me rolling my shoulders back and forth while tapping my foot and simultaneously tossing groceries onto the conveyer belt. She came over and put a gentle hand on my shoulder, mid-circuit.

Lisa took a business card out of her purse and handed it to me. It said, "Ivan Peptide, M.D., Neurology, Neurosurgery, Nervous Disorders."

"Call him," Lisa said. "He's really very, very good." She then smiled and as she walked away she said, "You don't have to live like this if you don't want to."

February 23

Last night, I dreamed about that chocolate trifle from Edie's party. I hadn't dreamed about food in years, since my last pregnancy. Was I losing my grip? But I couldn't get that trifle out of my mind. I wondered if Edie had any left. If she had, it would probably be going a little stale.

I didn't care. I called Edie, with the ostensible reason of wanting to thank her for the lovely party. Little did she know my true agenda! After congratulating her again on the anniversary and on the smashing festivities, I got down to business.

"That was some chocolate trifle you served the other night, Edie," I said. "I even broke my diet to eat some. It was *fabulous.*"

"Yes, wasn't it? I was so pleased with the caterer. Everybody seemed to enjoy the desserts."

"No doubt. Say, Edie, you wouldn't happen to have any of that trifle left, would you?"

"Why, yes, I do, as a matter of fact! I'm happy to give you what I've got, although, I must tell you that Lawrence had some last night and said it was getting a little hard around the edges."

"I'll take it," I said, too quickly. Imagine, stooping so low as to grovel for some hardened, stale trifle! Had I no self-respect anymore? I felt a need to redeem myself, if even a little. "Of course, I really shouldn't, since I'm trying to scrape off these pounds for the reunion, you know. But gee, it was really incredible."

"Oh, go ahead, if you liked it so much. Besides, there probably aren't as many calories in it now that it's going musty," Edie said. "Tell you what, I'm already going to be in your neighborhood on the way to the doctor this afternoon. I'll swing by and drop it off."

My God, she was even willing to make a house call. What could I say?

"Thanks, Edie, if you're really sure. . ."

"Absolutely! See you later!"

After we got off the phone, I thought about my friendship

with Edie. We had met as housemates in the Coop, long, long ago. I always suspected she had a passive-aggressive streak, and here it was again: She knew I shouldn't have any more of that trifle! Why was she willing to deliver it right to my door? We were about the same size; did she want to make sure the score stayed even? Of course, I did have options with the trifle. I could give it away. I could divvy it up for dessert to my family. I could throw it out. That's what any reputable diet advice would say about a situation like this. "Just throw out that leftover cake. Better in the garbage than on your hips!" How many times had I read nonsense like this? These are the same people who advise that if you have extra cookies on hand, divide the portions into small Baggies and put them in the freezer! As if I'm too stupid to figure out that I can just open the friggin' Baggie and eat the cookies frozen!

Unfortunately, I knew that I would not take any of these logical actions. After all, they demanded self-control, something I had in short supply these days. I knew that Edie would bring me the trifle and that furthermore, no one in the house would ever know about it.

February 24

I ate the leftover trifle. All of it. Then I got mad at Edie. So I called her again.

"Look, Edie, you knew I've been struggling with my weight. Why were you so quick to bring it over?"

"Hey, *you're* the one who asked for it. Besides, you must have been desperate to take it in *that* condition. I think you just needed a 'fix.' On the other hand, perhaps you need professional help. Have you considered Chocoholics Anonymous? Or a good therapist? I know an amazing one who specializes in food disorders."

"Edie, I *don't* have a food disorder. I just have an aversion to chronic hunger and prolonged chocolate deprivation. Besides, you know the old saying, 'Friends don't let friends eat leftover trifle.'"

"Listen, Judy, when you called, I had a choice to make: Either keep it in my refrigerator and probably eat it myself, or hand it over to you. Besides, even the closest of friendships can only go so far. Just do some extra exercise and you'll make up for it."

"Right. All I'll need to do is run from here to Iowa City and back, and all will be forgotten," I said.

Well, what's done is done. I did an extra half-hour exercise tape today, and vowed that next time we go to a party whose theme is desserts, I'm wearing a blindfold.

February 26

Last night I scared myself silly, and managed to aggravate Jeff at the same time. It was late, and we were getting ready for bed. I was tired from a long day, which included a tough Pilates routine, and couldn't wait to lie down. I got into bed, stretched out, and felt an alarming lump below my abdomen.

"Oh good God, a lump!" I said, first feeling one, and then immediately after, another. "Two! Something's wrong with me!" I wailed. Wasting no time, my overactive imagination immediately had me in the starring role of some two-hanky movie. Jeff ran out of the bathroom, still brushing his teeth, to see what was wrong. The lumps were strange, in that they were evenly spaced just above my pelvis. I felt a surge of self-pity. After working so hard and finally beginning to get in shape, could the end be near?

My husband ran to my side, looking pale. I showed him where I felt the lumps. He put his hand there, and then just shook his head.

"Those are your hip bones, you ninny!" he said.

I had hip bones? My gosh, come to think of it, they were in the correct place, a matching set. I don't think I had felt them since 1988. I leaped up out of bed and hugged him. "Thank God! I'm saved! Thank you, sweetheart!" I felt a surge of energy with the discovery of my new-found hip bones, available for detection by hand, if not yet by sight. The day ended well.

MARCH

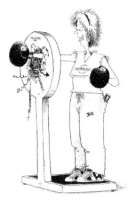

Belly Dancing, Boxing and the Bread of Affliction

March 3

At today's Weight Watchers meeting, the Scale of Injus tice reluc-tantly acknowledged that I had lost another pound. Carmen congratulated a woman for reaching her five-pound weight-loss milestone and another guy for los-ing his last ten.

"Yep, the first five and the last ten. Those are the hardest to lose," Carmen said. And then I realized: With fifteen pounds as my total weight loss goal, *every single blasted pound I had to lose was among the hardest!* Talk about depressing! Carmen also en-couraged us to ramp up our exercise, which was something I had learned a thing or two about. I raised my hand during this discussion to make what I felt a very pertinent point.

"You know muscle weighs more than fat, so even if you're

not losing a lot of pounds, you could still be getting a lot stronger and sleeker," I observed confidently, thinking about no one in particular.

"Yeah, well, that usually takes a long time," Carmen said, dissing my observation and dousing my enthusiasm. Well! The nerve! As a veteran Boot Camp warrior, budding Pilates powerhouse and home-based aerobicizer, I knew better, but I kept quiet. As I sat through the rest of the meeting, I calculated that it has now been sixty-two whole days since I have had any ice cream, and that if there was any fairness in the world, I would have lost more weight by now.

March 4

At the Rabbi's Roundtable today, Tanya shuffled in late, clutching a box of tissues. Her eyes were watery, and she coughed and sneezed frequently during the discussion about keeping the Sabbath. When class was over, I said to her, "I'm sorry you're not feeling well."

My aerobic training then proved its worth. Tanya sneezed violently and I was able to leap away with alacrity. Since I had started my own self-styled health regimen, I hadn't been sick once.

"I don't know what's the matter. I just can't shake this bug." Tanya looked at me with despair.

"My guess is that you're not getting enough zinc. You also may be biotin deficient," I said, feeling flush with knowledge.

"Look who's become an. . an. . AH- CHOOOO!" Tanya unleashed another geyser. ". . .an expert on health!" At that moment, she couldn't help but crack a smile. "You do look pretty healthy," she said.

"Never felt better," I told her. "I eat lots of dark, leafy vegetables, tofu, and salmon. And you were right about drinking water. It keeps the engine running smoothly, all right."

"Any other wisdom you'd like to share?" Tanya asked. I had her foggy attention.

"Just one little thing," I said. I then dug into my purse and extracted a miniature Hershey's Mr. Goodbar. "Of course you know that chocolate contains high levels of antioxidants known as polyphenols. And I find that a small bit of chocolate every day releases endorphins, which is a great mood enhancer. We all realize how crucial a positive mental attitude is for overall health."

"Thanks, Judy. I'll keep that in mind," she honked into a tissue.

I didn't mean to make Tanya feel worse. But it was *her* idea to eradicate sugar from her life. It wasn't too late for her to come back from the abyss.

March 5

When P.T. Barnum said, "There's a sucker born every minute," he clearly must have had someone like me in mind. The day had begun innocently enough, with me trying to select some new aerobics shoes in a sporting goods store. Now, this used to be a simple task, but has become so overwrought with overchoice that choosing a pair of sports shoes is much easier if you have, say, a degree in kineisiology. I became so befuddled by the choices among aerobic, cross-training, jogging, walking, and court shoes, I wandered away from the shoe department entirely and promptly fell into a marketing trap as wide as the Grand Canyon.

Between the yoga mats and the hand weights, I saw a whole slew of these silly looking ab-tightening belts that are the subject of just about every other infomercial on T.V. and selling faster than gym memberships in January. You power the thing up with some lithium batteries, strap it around your gut, thigh, chin, or whatever your main problem area seems to be, turn yourself on, and zap your fat away with electrical impulses. How stupid do these people think we are?

Of course, since the advertisements boasted that we could

"exercise" while lying around, watching the Leno show and eating nachos, I bought one. Despite many choices, including the "Flab-Slam," "AB-Be-Gone!" and "Slim-U-Later," I selected the "AB-Solution," perhaps because the model on the box looked as if he chewed iron for breakfast. I tried to hold my head high while placing the device on the counter to pay and noticed the clerk tightly pursing her mouth, in an effort to keep from laughing directly in my face.

I was very eager to start electrocuting my fat away, so when I came home I popped the instructional video in the television immediately. I then was greeted on the video by a specimen of physical perfection named Hilly, a name that aptly described her chest, if not her intellect. Hilly announced her credentials to teach me about the AB-Solution by saying that she was a Certified Fitness Instructor. Based on her complexion, which, if I had to give it a name would call it "Science Fiction Bronze," I gathered that she gave all her fitness classes in a tanning salon booth.

Hilly and the AB-Solutions manufacturer must have guessed that the only doofuses who would buy this contraption had the mental acuity of a potato, because Hilly made sure to speak v-e-r-y s-l-o-w-l-y, and even felt it necessary to offer visual cues. For example, when Hilly spoke about herself, she pointed to herself, and then, very helpfully, pointed to the camera to indicate when we were being spoken to. To avoid any other misunderstandings, Hilly also pointed to her hips when she meant hips, abdomen when she meant abdomen, and thighs when she meant thighs.

As Hilly explained how we were to apply the "slimming gel" on the belt, we were treated to video shots of other impossibly fit, gorgeous couples as they washed their cars or cooked their low-carb dinners, all while wearing their AB-Solution belts. They were, of course, smiling and in love. "Yes, you too can get in shape, *without breaking a sweat!*" Hilly claimed, s-l-o-w-l-y. As with any diet plan, though, Hilly warned that consistency was the key. To have any chance of ever looking like her, we needed to use the AB-Solution each day, in each problem area, haul ourselves off the couch for some real physical exertion every week or so, remember never to throw the AB-Solution belt (which was constructed of the finest materials) into the washing machine, and also to take the specially formulated nutritional supplements that came with the belt. These were a lot of instructions for doofuses to remember.

Before she actually showed us how to use the belt for the first time, Hilly suggested we stop the video and call the toll-free number to order MORE lithium batteries, MORE slimming gel and MORE supplements, so as to "maximize results," undoubtedly those of her company's profits. By this point, though, I was getting antsy, as the kids were due home soon, and I sure hoped to get in a good ten-minute electronic workout before they did. I was ready to see if, as Hilly said, the AB-Solution would really change my life!

Thanks to Hilly's crack teaching skills, I learned that the "plus sign" on the batteries indicated "positive," and the "minus sign" indicated "negative," though she used one-syllable words and other hand motions to impart this knowledge. I snapped in my batteries, just as Hilly told me to, and smeared myself with the gel, the kind they use when doing ultrasound.

I velcroed the belt around my midsection, turned on the power switches, and waited to see my washboard abs break out from captivity. Just my luck, though, only one of the two power units worked! I wondered if, sensing the big job ahead of it, the other power unit simply blew a fuse. I did feel a slight tingling sensation, but couldn't imagine that this would do much, so after a few minutes, I started pressing the power button again repeatedly to maximize the intensity. Soon, I was at full power! I felt I could launch a NASA booster rocket! I walked around the house, with the shades drawn, and tried to go about my business, while my new AB-Solution belt was zapping my fat in a two-inch radius into oblivion. I had to remove the belt repeatedly and add more gel before rotating the one working power unit, to target other areas. It was getting messy.

Then, unexpectedly, I heard the front door open. The kids were home! All I was wearing was a pair of exercise shorts, a bra and the AB-Solution belt! I quickly ran to my room, still vibrating at full throttle. I shut the door, and heard the clarion call, "MOM!"

I opened my bedroom door a crack and shouted, "There's nobody here by that name!" and slammed the door. By this time, I couldn't take much more stimulation, so I turned myself off, wiped off the gel from the belt and my belly, and got dressed.

While still hiding from the kids, I carefully read the ingredients and instructions on the nutritional supplement that came with the belt. It contained something called "Hyper-Meta-Phedra-Bolic," a compound so powerful it needed four inches of minuscule-size type to warn us of all its potential side effects. Using a microscope, I read the warning: "Hyper-Meta-Phedra-Bolic is a completely safe and natural product which may, in some individuals, result in unnatural reactions. Not intended for use by individuals with a history of heart disease, seizures, high blood pressure, low blood pressure, any blood pressure, toothaches, bellyaches, bunions, and annoying in-laws. Not intended to replace food. Contraindicated for individuals taking any medication of any kind, including breath mints. Stop taking this supplement immediately if you have a heart attack." I called to cancel my order for a six-month supply.

Not only am I afraid of Hyper-Meta-Phedra-Bolic, but something tells me that even if I wore the AB-Solution belt all day, I'm never going to look like Hilly. And then there's the potential unknown risk that even if I did use the belt as directed, I might end up *sounding* like her. I think I'll return the AB-Solution tomorrow. I need to go back anyway to devote at least three hours to further study of the vast universe of exercise shoes.

March 7

Kate threw herself a birthday party and invited a belly dancer to come and give a lesson. I thought this was a stroke of genius, a clever way to work off all the desserts we had been devouring beforehand. While cleaning off a plate of cream cheese-filled brownies, it occurred to me that belly dancing would be a good supplement to my exercise routine. After all, it would be hard to get bored with something so exotic!

The next day, I called the dancer, Hypnotica, and told her I wanted to sign up for her next class.

"Beginning, intermediate, or advanced?" she asked.

I thought about this. The most exotic dancing I had done in recent years was thrusting my right hip to slam the dryer shut while balancing a basket of laundry on my left, a move perfected after years of repetition. "Beginning," I said.

Hypnotica sounded very excited to meet me, perhaps unnaturally so, but I took down the address and committed to be there.

"What should I wear?" I asked, suddenly realizing that my belly-dancing wardrobe was a little sparse.

"Oh, a skirt, a scarf, whatever you feel comfortable with," she said airily. Was that all, I wondered? How was I to allocate these few garments on my body? I was afraid to ask.

After pawing through my closet and finding my most bewitching accessory to be an aging sweatband, I showed up at class wearing regular workout clothes. I was appalled to find that the other women in the class were decked out in low-slung sequined skirts and beaded halter tops, revealing abs so flat I wanted to dance my belly right out of the studio. To distract myself, I ran around the room, which faced the street, shutting all the blinds. These gals may be happy to let the public watch them urge their hips around, as if we were performing at a cabaret, but I had not yet achieved this level of professionalism.

Hypnotica looked fetching in a gold mesh skirt fringed with coins and matching halter also dripping with sequins. She wore a heavy silver choker and enough bracelets to anchor a cruise ship. She popped in the CD, filling the room with Middle Eastern music. I felt myself instantly transported to Cairo, and even thought I smelled cardamom and curry.

"Are you ready?" Hypnotica asked in a throaty voice, tossing back her mane of long black hair. She looked at me, sashayed over and asked, "Tell me, can you roll your belly at all?"

"Sure. Just say something funny."

"Ah, you are humorous, I see!" Hypnotica said. "Never mind. We will get to that later." She then led us in some stretches, and then put her hands on her hips. "Now, feel your hips, feel the power of your femininity!"

I placed my hands on my hips, and tried to focus on this suggestion. Come to think of it, I did recall many instances when this area of my anatomy had indeed proven to be my main power base: planting them against the door to keep a child in time-out, balancing a shoulder roast on one hip while slinging a pot of hot pasta into the colander, carting children on one hip until I ached and needed to switch them to the other side. Oh yes, and then there was that small matter of giving birth. Four times, only one of which included painkillers of any kind. I'll never forgive the natural childbirth movement. What kind of sadists were they?

Hypnotica's goal for this first class was to teach us to gyrate our center of femininity around while keeping our head and shoulders completely still. We were to imagine a total separation between hips and upper abdomen. This would take practice, she assured us, and encouraged us in our movements, no matter how spastic they appeared. As I gyrated, my bones registered their protest by making all kinds of embarrassing snapping and groaning sounds. Other than Hypnotica, I was the oldest woman in the room, and felt just slightly younger than the Pyramids. It was possible that I was past my belly-dancing prime.

Watching myself in the mirror, I began to wonder whether I should try something else physically challenging but where elaborate costumes were not mandatory. Given my experience as a stay-at-home mother, I thought about becoming a waitress or UPS delivery person. The prospect of my wearing spangled tops and wrap skirts sent a shudder down my spine, but UPS brown was a nice neutral color that went with everything. However, I was getting into the groove of the music and the movement. Before I realized it, Hypnotica had us all doing the "camel," a dance where we made circular arcs with our shoulders and then our hips. I concentrated hard on emulating the camel, and in the process realized I had never given this animal proper credit for moving so artfully. To think I had taken it for granted! It was humbling to feel less elegant than a camel, but at least I had better teeth.

I was still doing my camel impersonation, jutting my chest forward while arcing my hips back, and was even prepared to have someone sling a fifty-pound sack of spices on my back and say "giddy up!" or whatever one says to camels, when Hypnotica came over to me and pointed out that the session was over.

"You did a wonderful job for your first time," she said to me. "You were so . . . " (here she seemed to struggle for the right word) "*fearless!* You simply didn't care *how* you looked when you danced, you just celebrated your femininity! I see a lot of potential." I tried to look humble. Maybe I wasn't past my prime after all.

March 11
(six pounds down on my scale)

I am *this close* to getting my five-pound bookmark from Weight Watchers! I lost another 1.4 pounds at today's weigh-in, which made me so happy that I began to form plans to splurge on a raspberry danish after the meeting. After all, it was Lawrence Welk's birthday and the day of the American Bowling Congress Convention and Hall of Fame Induction Ceremonies. The bad news, at least according to them, was that I had skipped the last two meetings, and they wanted to charge me even for those!

"You already used up all your free 'skipped' meetings," Carmen told me. "On the plan you're on, you can only miss three meetings before having to pay for skipped meetings."

"But that's not fair! How can you possibly charge me for *not* coming to a meeting?" I was a little incensed, especially since at that moment they were running my credit card through the machine, not only for the cost of today's meeting but also for several boxes of chocolate crisp two-point bars. Dastardly deeds had been done somewhere in the corporate office, and they had discontinued my favorite flavor, the chocolate mint bars. Now I'll have to search for them on the black market. In any case, it was impossible for me to have gone to the last two meetings. One Sunday I forgot to set the alarm. And last Sunday, I was out of town for business, something I had precious little time for these days, what with all this exercising, water drinking Olympiads, carpooling, taking the hamsters to the vet, helping one kid decorate his display board for his social studies report on Micronesia, and trying to minimize the damage caused by one child's self-inflicted haircut.

"Hey, don't you realize what a *bargain* this is?" Carmen asked, incredulous. "You know how much it would cost you just to walk in the doors of Lindora or Jenny Craig? At the cheap rate you pay, if we didn't have this rule people would just come and go as they pleased. Remember, Weight Watchers is a *commitment.*"

Carmen recommended that I switch to a more expensive plan, which costs fourteen bucks per meeting, but I'd only need to come once a month before they sent a posse after me. I recognized a danger here immediately. Without the specter of a Sunday weigh-in hanging over my head every week, I'd probably revert to my slothful ways for three weeks out of the month and then show up at the end of the month six pounds heavier. The honchos at Weight Watchers had my number, all right. I told her I'd think about it.

Still, our group was smashingly successful today. The woman in charge of the scales ran up to Carmen in the middle of the meeting, after she tallied the flesh of all latecomers, and handed her a note.

Carmen looked at it and exclaimed, "Hey, guys, you lost 97.8 pounds this week! *Waytago!*" We all applauded our thinner selves, and as I looked around, the room really did seem a little airier.

It's hard to pinpoint the major highlight of today's meeting. At first it seemed to be the moment when the woman sitting in front of me stood up to accept her official Weight Watchers anchor-themed key chain for losing ten percent of her body fat. We were appropriately humbled by this feat, and while I applauded, I couldn't help but wonder: an anchor? Was this the appropriate symbol for such a Herculean achievement? Why not a glazed donut, with a big red slash line through it? Or a salad bowl, brimming with antioxidant-filled, zero-point vegetables?

But after we finished oohing and aahing over today's heroic flab-fighters, a sudden dispute arose over egg whites that had every one of us on the edge of our seats. A woman who looked as if she had no reason to be at Weight Watchers posed a question to Carmen that started the whole uproar. She asked, "If two egg whites have zero points, but three egg whites have one point, can you eat two egg whites at 8:00 a.m. and another two egg whites at 11:00 a.m. and still count it as zero points?" This is the type of Talmudic hair-splitting that goes on in Weight Watchers meetings, and I for one felt sorry for anyone who was too dumb to realize that the only eggs worth eating were ones that included at least one yolk. What was she saving up all her points for, anyway? A bag of carrots?

Still, the great egg white debate got a lot of people exercised, and political factions began sprouting up around the room: the one-pointers versus the zero-pointers. Of course, I cast my vote with the zero pointers, because I am always lenient in these matters. Because of our involvement with the big egg controversy, however, people lost interest in the other activity we had been engaged in, which was passing an onion around the room. As we held it, we were to imagine that the onion was really a potato and then guess how many points it would have. I'm going to try to remember this the next time I throw a party and things get dull. As it turned out, few people realize how much potato you can really eat for only four points. (Conversely, few people realize that merely being in the same room with a large cinnamon bun costs you four points. Looking at the cinnamon bun is eight points, thinking illicit thoughts about it is twelve. Eating it costs about thirty points, so I can kiss those buns goodbye – that's more than a full day's allotment for me!)

Carmen, who eventually voted with the one-pointers, calmed the excited crowd by segueing to her final instruction to us, which was the importance of "journaling," or writing everything down in our diaries. I looked at mine, and it was alarmingly clean. I was always good about journaling on Sundays, after the meeting, but I tended to trail off and lose track of the diary, not to mention what I was eating, by Tuesday. But since I am so close to getting my bookmark, I am going to be really careful this week.

March 17 (down seven pounds, though Weight Watchers disagrees)

I've learned a very important lesson today. And that is, when I am retaining more water than the Hoover Dam and have chosen to wear my t-shirt that says, "I've Got PMS. . . And I've Got a Gun!" I should just skip the Weight Watchers meeting. And yet, I was so good this week, only a half-pound away from my five-pound milestone and bookmark! I wanted my bookmark! I wanted to be among the few, the proud, the brave, who finally got to raise their hands when Carmen asked, "Did anybody achieve their five-pound weight loss today?" That should have been ME!

I got on the scale and sensed trouble immediately when the scale simply could not settle down. The numbers kept jumping all over the place, as if the scale was having a nervous breakdown.

"Hey, what gives?" I asked, as the weigher-inner and I simply stared in disbelief at the jumpy digital numbers. The scale probably had repetitive stress injury – who could blame it? But I found it insulting nonetheless. I got off and got on again, and the scale eventually stabilized at a number that put me *up* by half a pound. I was crestfallen. But more than that, I was *mad!*

I grabbed my weigher-inner by her Weight Watchers pin that said, "I lost 39 pounds in 2001" and said with gritted teeth, "This isn't just! This isn't fair! This is just *water retention!*" I sensed that people were staring at me.

She gently removed my hand from her person, read my t-shirt and took a step back. "Let's see," she said, in an exaggeratedly calm tone that one uses when speaking to the mentally deranged, "Take off your glasses." I did, but with no weight-loss effect. She then suggested I go use the bathroom. Did she think I was that stupid? I had already tried that and every other trick in the book, including having clipped my fingernails and toe nails that morning. She then told me to remove my watch, my earrings, my wedding ring. We might as well have been playing strip poker. The crowds were getting restless outside the booth – this weigh-in was taking a long time. Unfortunately, I was not so heavily weighed down with gold and other precious metals that removing my jewelry made any difference in the final tally according to that crazy scale.

My weigher-inner oozed low-calorie sympathy and encouraged me to come back next week, when I was certain to have lost the water weight. She even said that, all things considered, a half-pound up "during this time" was pretty darned good.

I sat down in a foul mood. Carmen's first topic today was stress, and how it can hamper the digestive system. I tell you, sometimes it seems as if you're damned no matter what you do! And, speaking of digestive disorders, she also spoke about the coming Passover and Easter holidays and tips for surviving them in a Weight Watchers world. She noted that as a Jew, she could not muster much sympathy for the Easter celebrants, who only had one festive meal and a few chocolate bunnies to contend with, whereas Jews had eight days of heavy Passover meals, including several full-fledged feasts celebrating the Exodus from Egypt. Now that I think about it, no wonder it took us forty years of wandering in the desert before coming to the Promised Land. It had to have taken that long just to walk off all that matzah.

I was so upset by today's weigh-in that it took all my powers of self-control, pathetic as they are, not to stop at the market and get a jumbo-sized Hershey's bar, which I believe even doctors recommend as an emergency substitute for Prozac. However, I did try a new kind of soy nutrition bar that boasted among its ingredients twenty-four essential vitamins and minerals and a dedication to saving the rainforest.

I found it tasted really good with chocolate syrup.

March 19 (103 days before Coop reunion)

The reunion is only three months away and I am only down by seven lousy pounds on my scale, and not quite five pounds on the Weight Watchers scale. Not only that, next week begins eight days of eating dry, nearly indigestible matzah, the aptly named "bread of affliction." How will I survive so many big holiday meals, filled with meat, wine, and matzah? Despite these hurdles, I'm determined to go back to Weight Watchers next week even though I will just have completed a marathon of three days of holiday eating, and collect my bookmark.

It will be nearly remarkable if I can pull it off. Even Carmen said she expects to gain weight over Passover. But I am determined to get to reach this milestone, matzah ball soup or no matzah ball soup (and I suspect it will have to be the latter). To help achieve this lofty goal, today I took a Latin dance class at The Sculpted Self, where I took a tour and got a week's pass. I had vowed to stay away from gyms altogether after my unhappy encounters at Muscle Mart and Bodies by Barbarella, but I'm no quitter. I worried at first when I walked in The Sculpted Self and saw dozens of bucko guys with snarling looks on their faces hefting hundreds of pounds of weights, but most of these he-men were at least more normally proportioned than those thundering, overbulked bruisers I had seen at Muscle Mart. Who knows? Maybe these guys were Muscle Mart rejects!

I admit I was a bit surprised to be greeted at The Sculpted Self by a short, squat guy sitting at a desk and depositing a double cheeseburger and triple order of fries into a swag belly the size of a bay window. Involved as he was in bolting down his burger, he seemed reluctant to stand up all the way to greet me, but waved me in cheerfully. "Wannalookaround?" he asked, his mouth full of burger.

The man, Luigi, swept his food to the side, creating a fry-free zone on his desk, and beckoned me to sit down. Between swallows of fast food, this startling representative of the fitness industry extolled the virtues of the gym, and then pulled out a notebook with the printed fees for club membership. These included a confusing array of payment plans, including one where I could pay several thousand dollars up front, but this would get me paid up three years in advance and include validated parking.

"I just came to look around and get the free week's pass advertised in the newspaper," I said, not having a spare several thousand dollars on me.

Luigi, who bore an uncanny resemblance to Danny DeVito, paused for a moment, sizing up the situation. "I got no problem with that. But let me just tell you that if you join right now, *today*," (here he ripped a piece of paper from a pad and whipped a pen out with a dramatic flourish) "I can offer you a club membership at this *unbelievable* price." He then wrote down a number much smaller than any printed in the notebook, a number that he probably made up on the spot. His expression seemed to defy me to find a comparably generous offer anywhere in the universe of fitness clubs. Luigi then leaned close to me and said in a slightly conspiratorial tone that he had heard that Bodies by Barbarella would soon be going bankrupt, and that hundreds, maybe even thousands of Barbarella's refugees would soon be storming the locker rooms of The Sculpted Self. When that happened, I couldn't possibly expect him to make the same offer.

"That's understandable, but I'd really like to try a few classes first, make sure the music doesn't destroy my hearing or my spirit. Then, if I like the classes, I'll join. But I would like to get my pass."

"I got no problem with that," Luigi said, finally hauling himself up and showing me many of the club's features, such as individual television screens on the exercise equipment. After touring three dozen machines that toned every possible area of anatomy, including some I had never heard of, I asked if we could go upstairs to see the main classroom.

"I got no problem with that," said Luigi, apparently at a loss for more innovative conversational patterns. As I headed toward the stairs, he said, "C'mon, the elevator's right here. Save your energy for the classes, know what I mean?" He chuckled.

"I got no problem with that, Luigi," I said.

Upstairs, Luigi proudly stroked a display of hand weights, as if he had personally cast each and every one of them. "Beautiful, aren't they?"

I agreed that they were. He pointed out the new sticky yoga mats, the full-sized step platforms, and the new punching bags, which he reminded me were a convenient way to work out any pent-up hostility I felt towards any members of my family or society at large. He then unleashed a bit of his own hostility on one unsuspecting bag, just for good measure, and then smiled at me. Finally, he dared me to go into the ladies' locker room and then come out and tell him if it wasn't a clean enough suite in which to perform open-heart surgery.

"It's a marvel of housekeeping maintenance, Luigi," I said, and he nodded with pride.

After completing the tour, which also included an office with full chiropractic services, body fat testing, and a little store where one could purchase protein powder in canisters the size of grain silos, I finally squeezed Luigi for the free pass. I made my escape, barely making it in time for the Latin dance class.

Jennifer, the teacher, was terrific. I had never taken Latin dance before, but found my previous belly dancing training came in handy, since most of the moves involved hip thrusting of some kind or another. And I could do it! When Jennifer called out, "C'mon! Give me some HIPS!" I was thrilled. After all, looking around the room it was obvious that I had more to give in this department than anyone else. I didn't understand the lyrics, since they were all in Spanish, but I got the "Ole, ole, ole!" part. Based on some of the other modern lyrics I have heard in what passes for English these days, I'm probably better off *not* having understood the rest.

Now, from a calorie burning standpoint, Latin dance had it all over belly dancing. Not only that, I didn't need to wear two-dozen bracelets or itty-bitty scarves tied around my center point of femininity to participate. Enough attention gravitated to that area naturally. I did not need special effects.

At the end of class, I thanked Jennifer, who complimented me on my dancing abilities.

"Well, I *have* had some experience belly dancing, and that really helps, you know," I said, trying to appear modest.

Jennifer was duly impressed.

Finally, a little respect.

March 26

My knuckles are not nearly so swollen anymore, but they are still a horrendous purplish-green and a bit puffy. This is my reward for listening to the wisdom of Luigi, who assured me that I'd be fine trying the Extreme Cardio-Box class one time without the gloves, conveniently sold in an assortment of primary colors just outside the classroom. I wasn't yet ready to commit to buying a pair, so I commandeered Jeff's ski gloves as a minor form of protection and sneaked them into my gym bag before leaving the house. I was not about to tell the family that I was going out to box, knowing full well they'd snicker at me. By now they are so used to my dashing out the door with gym bag in hand that they have stopped asking if it's yoga, step-cardio or Boot Camp night. I have managed to keep the belly dancing a secret from my daughter, since it would hardly do to have her spread all over school that her mother belly dances.

I felt ridiculous wearing Jeff's ski gloves when the thirty-five other Extreme-Cardio Boxers in class had encased their fists in the real thing, but I am used to feeling ridiculous by now. After all, I'm the woman who always brought up the rear in Boot Camp, jangled like Fort Knox at belly dancing class and twisted myself into pretzel shapes at yoga from which I was only extricated when the paramedics came and used the "Jaws of Life."

I was surprised that the instructor was a lithe little thing named Mandy. She couldn't have been more than five feet tall and 105 pounds sopping wet. But when I watched her nimbly demonstrate an upper right hook and roundhouse kick, I knew it would be a mistake for anyone to take a fling at this featherweight!

Considering that I loathe, despise, detest and in every other way abhor boxing, I couldn't believe how much fun I had in class. Mandy was all business, though. We started with a bracing series of jumping jacks, then jogged around the room, weaving in and out of each punching bag. At our punching bags we practiced jabs, kicks, punching and ducking, and even that funny little ballet step I've only seen when I was forced to see a few minutes of a real boxing match. It was a great workout, and I gave it my all, especially since I didn't realize all the damage I was doing to my poor hands, which still had a dozen Passover meals to shop and cook for. I remembered what Luigi said about using the punching bags to work the pent-up hostility out of my system, and discovered I had more of it than I realized. For example, I thought about having been in the telephone purgatory of "hold" that morning with the phone company, listening to their voice recording repeating its mantra that "my call was very important to them. Please stay on the line for the next available operator." I remained in this purgatory for forty-two minutes (I clocked it) until a real person finally got on the line. Then we got cut off. UPPER RIGHT HOOK!

I thought about my children's behavior in the car after school, during which they proved once again that no topic under the sun, including a discussion of what day of the week it really was, was too trivial for a fight. I pleaded with them to just settle down, a call I had repeated more times than the phone company has ever had to assure its customers that their calls are very important to them. And I thought about the package of potato chips they fought over in the back seat until the package broke and potato chips went flying around the van, ushering in screams of outrage from all parties involved. ROUNDHOUSE KICK!

Since I was already all worked up, I recalled being in the supermarket that day in line behind a woman who insisted on excavating her purse for that last coupon that she just knew was in there. She took such an agonizingly long time, I was sure that either she or the coupon would expire by the time she found it. Meanwhile, I had exactly fourteen minutes to check out, load the car, race home, unload the bags and dash to school to pick up the kids so they wouldn't be late for karate. But this was a woman determined not to let a twenty-cent coupon stand between her and six angry customers behind her. By the time she gave up and paid, she counted out her single dollar bills and rolls of nickels so slowly I thought I would scream. JAB! JAB! UPPER LEFT HOOK!

Should I be alarmed that my favorite exercises so far are either militaristic or pugilistic in nature? I think not. Instead, I'm focusing on the happy observation that many of my clothes are getting too big!

Filled with adrenaline after my first session with Mandy's boxing class, I also knuckled under and bought a membership at The Sculpted Self. The commission Luigi earned for signing me up made us fast friends, although I daresay not as fast as he is with a drive-through order at Wendy's.

March 29

I did it! After three days of straight eating, punctuated by going to synagogue and praying that I wouldn't gain weight, I went to Weight Watchers this morning, weighed in wearing the lightest little cotton frock I owned, and miraculously lost another half-pound, thus achieving my five-pound milestone! So, now that the hardest first five pounds were gone, all I had left were the hardest last ten pounds!

I still suspect that something is off about the scales at Weight Watchers. I *know* I had lost two pounds before I began the program to begin with, but I was happy regardless. And at the last meeting, two of the scales even conked out, and Carmen was reduced to asking if anyone had any batteries handy!

Carmen had made a big deal warning us not to be too disappointed if we gained weight from the holidays, and even she confessed to having gained three pounds, so I felt a little smug because I hadn't. I can't really understand how I did it, either. True, I had passed up the richest foods and kugels, but I had not denied myself my special date-chocolate Passover cake. I can only guess that many calories were burned while shopping, cleaning, boxing, cooking and serving food endlessly for days and days. That, and God must have thrown His mercy on me. He had, I'm sure, helped me earn my bookmark, even if I only made it by one ounce.

While Carmen droned on about always being prepared with a two-point bar or some other low-point snack in case of sudden and acute hunger, I just sat there impatiently until my big moment. Finally she asked for a show of hands from people who had lost weight. My hand shot up like a rocket.

"C'mon up here and accept your five-pound bookmark!" Carmen invited.

With a blush on my slimmer face, I rose from my seat and sidled my way through the thick crowd to the front of the room. Sucking in my not-yet-firm abs, I accepted my bookmark from Carmen and looked out at the sea of my fellow congregants at Weight Watchers, nodding humbly to their enthusiastic applause. There is nothing wrong with a token amount of public adulation, I thought, gripping my paper bookmark with greater pride than I had felt when I accepted the sheepskin at graduation from the U. nearly twenty years earlier.

In celebration, I finished off the last bits of the date cake later that afternoon. It was time to clean out the pan, anyway.

APRIL

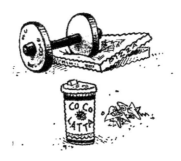

Guru Hari and the Forty Thieves

April 1

I was excited to return to Boot Camp last night, where I hadn't been for a long time. I hoped the Major would notice my improved, streamlined appearance, but if he didn't, I planned to point it out to him.

"Private Gruen! Good to see you!" the Major greeted me.

"Hoo Yah, Major! Good to be back."

"How long has it been now?"

"Two months, but I haven't been idle, sir. Don't you notice that I look slimmer?" I couldn't believe I had said that. What had happened to my self-respect and dignity? Had it been burned up with some fat?

"Yep, you sure do, but let's see how you can keep up tonight. It's going to be a tough session."

These military men! So hard to please!

At the stroke of six o'clock, the Major blew his whistle

and we began our run. He started alongside me and said, "Okay, little miss 'I think I'll miss two months of Boot Camp.' Now pick up the pace and show me what you've got!"

I never like to disappoint the Major, so I ran as fast as my short legs could carry me without having to call upon his training as a paramedic. We sang one of my favorite cadences, with the Major singing each line and the rest of us repeating after him:

> C-130 rolling down the strip,
> Boot Camp Warrior on a one-way trip.
> Mission top secret, destination unknown.
> We don't even know if we'll ever come home.
> Stand up, hook up, shuffle to the door.
> Jump on out and count to four.
> If my main don't open wide,
> I've got a reserve by my side.
> If that one don't fail me too,
> Look out below, I'm a comin' through!
> If I land in a puddle of mud,
> Bury me with a case of Bud!
> A case of Bud and a bottle of rum,
> and we'll raise hell till the kingdom come.
> Pin my medals upon my chest,
> and bury me in the leaning rest.
> Tell my mom I'd done my best,
> Meet St. Peter at the pearly gates.
> Oh no, I'm a little late.
> When I get to heaven, St. Peter's gonna say,
> How'd you earn your livin? How'd you earn your pay?
> And I will reply with a little bit of anger:
> Earned my livin' as a Boot Camp Warrior!
> Boot camp Warrior!
> Body fat destroyer!
> Motivated!
> Dedicated!
> Armor plated!
> Always wet, never dry
> We never sleep and that's no lie.
> Hoo-yah!
> Hoo-yah!

I was happy to be reunited with the other recruits. And I was thrilled to rise to the Major's challenge. Last winter, I could only sing a few lines of our cadences before running out of breath. I was not capable, as it were, of running and singing at the same time. No more. Tonight I sang every line, while not missing a beat on the run! Realizing how much more stamina I had made me run even faster. The Major even told me to slow down at one point. Ha! Who ever would have thunk it? It is a grave mistake to ever underestimate the power and determination of a Jewish mother.

The only impediment to Boot Camp bliss was Allison. She was a lively and friendly enough fellow warrior, but she vexed me greatly when she started griping about the harsh unfairness of not being able to lose weight proportionate to her stick-thin figure. Even back in January, Allison was yapping that she just got "too skinny" around the waist, while her hips remained, gee, I don't know, thirty-one or thirty-two inches around. Now it was April, she was as scrawny as ever and still mewling about this gross inequity. Two other warriors and I, more amply built than waif-like Allison, just gritted our teeth and squeezed each other's shoulders to keep us from belting Allison in her skinny face. She babbled on, oblivious to the blow she was delivering to troop morale.

The rest of our session entailed grueling push-ups, leg lifts, sit-ups, sprints up and down stairs, and more running. I complimented some of the other recruits, telling them how well they looked. They did, but I was also fishing for compliments for myself at the same time. I really did not want to have to resort to pointing out the obvious to everybody, namely, that there was a little less of me than there had been back at the end of January. However, no one commented on this development.

Really, some people can become so self-absorbed.

April 3

Now that I'm a member of The Sculpted Self, I am planning to get my money's worth. This grew to be a slightly larger task today when I got a parking ticket on the street near the club. I suppose it was my fault, not bringing my magnifying glass to read the fine print on the highest of the four street signs posted, one pegged on top of the other, indicating the few measly hours that the city deemed it allowable for the tax-paying citizenry to park on public streets. The relevant sign did state that I could have parked there if it had been a Sunday between two a.m. and seven-forty-five a.m., unless it was a full moon or Martin Luther King's birthday. It would have taken me a half-hour to decipher all the other warnings, and so I dashed off in pursuit of health and well being. To add insult to injury, I could have parked in the gym's underground garage for free, but as I am living a health-conscious lifestyle, I purposefully walked from a few blocks away. No one can accuse me of only "talking the talk." I am also "walking the walk," though it is getting a little pricey.

There are few things I hate more than parking tickets, with the possible exception of the oxymoron "customer service" and people who slap vapid bumper stickers on their cars that say "Visualize World Peace" but who offer only an extremely rude hand gesture if you ask them to please let you into their lane so you can make a left turn. Of course, they never do, presumably because they are too busy visualizing world peace, which must be breaking out in another galaxy. I have always believed that parking meters are an affront to democracy, and I sure wish someone would take up this cudgel and fight to eradicate them, like they are doing with land mines. I'd do it myself except that I am too busy trying to become fit and fabulous after forty, which has become darned near a full-time job.

However, today I discovered something else that I hate as much as I do these other things, and that is a nutty exercise called spinning. I always thought spinning sounded like something you did with yarn or a top, not the human body. Curious about the craze, I once asked a spinning instructor, whom I had met at a women's retreat, what the big deal was.

"Isn't this just a marketing term to describe riding a stationary bicycle?" I asked her. She looked at me as if I had just told her that her first-born was ugly. Grabbing my wrist, she looked at me fiercely and said, "Spinning will *change your life!*"

That sounded like an awfully big promise to me, and her militancy on the subject scared me. Now that I am working to get fighting trim, though, I was ready to give it a chance. However, my original instincts proved right. Spinning is basically forty-five minutes of hell on stationary wheels.

Parking so far away had already cost me precious minutes of calorie-busting, and I came to class late. After running upstairs, I saw that everyone was pedaling as if their lives depended on it. They looked as if they were racing the Tour De France, only they weren't going anywhere, and had no Evian water waiting for them at the finish. I brought a bike out from the corner of the room and then looked in my bag for my gym shoes. Blast! I had forgotten them in the car! I was wearing platform sandals, a completely ridiculous type of footgear for spinning, but I wasn't going to waste any more time, so I just hopped on the bike and tried to pedal.

Immediately I realized something was wrong, and it wasn't only my absurd shoes. Not only was the seat really uncomfortable, but when I tried to pedal, I felt as if I were pushing against a Sherman tank. How could everyone else be going so fast? Despite the noxious and deafening music crucifying my ear drums and tormenting my soul, I noticed a friendly lady on the bike next to me signaling me to boost my seat higher and lower the bike's resistance. Aha! It took me a few moments to disentangle my clunky sandals from the foot harness and dismount the bike, but I followed her instructions. Even so, I had had enough after five minutes. If I thought being on hold with the phone company was purgatory, at least I could have a cup of coffee while enduring it. This, truly, was mind-bogglingly boring, and my legs gave out alarmingly fast.

I couldn't believe all these people were doing this willingly. I looked around and was gratified to see that most folks appeared somewhat miserable, though not nearly as much as I thought appropriate under the circumstances. Some really got excited, even whooping and shouting, when the teacher commanded us to set the resistance higher, and pick up our fannies to ride in a different, though still tortuous, manner. But no one was enjoying the class as much as Cindy, the teacher, who sang karaoke to the staccato howling blasting through the CD player. During another atonal auditory barrage, Cindy appeared to be in the throes of passion and bore an expression that I found embarrassing. She must have had her bike on a different setting than mine.

To protect myself from having a heart attack, I took frequent breaks, during which I mulled over this crazy scene: so many healthy people, living in a climate-controlled city on a beautiful, smog-free spring day, all pedaling their kishkes out in a sweaty room on bikes going nowhere. Only in Los Angeles, I thought!

When the class was over, the woman who tried to help me with my bike said, "You must be new here."

"How'd you guess?"

"It's hard for everyone at the beginning. And you kept the resistance on your bike much too high. And another thing," she added, "next time bring aerobics shoes."

I didn't want her to think I was totally witless, and began to follow her to explain. But she bounded down the stairs so quickly, and my legs were so wobbly, I couldn't catch her. I felt like Gumby, as I went down the stairs very, very slowly, enfeebled by my session on that wretched bike.

When I got to the car, I ripped the parking ticket from my windshield and went home, feeling a headache coming on.

April 5

The other night, after the spinning debacle, my headache mushroomed into a walloping migraine, the kind best dealt with through general anesthesia. I could not bear any light, could not bear anybody or anything, and simply buried myself under a blanket on the couch, moaning piteously. Some member of my family, fatigued by my bellyaching, managed to haul me off to bed for the night.

The next morning, Jeff had diagnosed the problem. "Never go to that spinning class again!" he warned, as I was nursing a cup of very high-octane coffee to help me to feel vaguely human again. "It had to have been that music you told me they played in there. It damages the psyche."

"You can't necessarily blame the spinning class," I said, though I dearly wanted to, so I would have a reason never to return. However, I felt it only fair to try any exercise class twice before renouncing it for life. "Say, did you know that a whole cup of fat-free cottage cheese has only two points? I can eat all this and a mango and still have a small cookie for only five points. That's a good deal."

"Hrmmm."

"Did you say something?"

"No. It's just that I really don't need to know the point value of everything you put in your mouth. Were you interested in knowing the point value of the refinanced mortgage I was telling you I might get for the house? Now *that's* important."

"I thought you might be proud of me for becoming more disciplined and for working to get in better shape. Some husbands would appreciate that in a wife who is approaching the age of a fine wine."

Jeff snapped the newspaper shut. "I thought you looked fine in the first place, and I'm glad you're getting in shape. But really, you're not half the woman you used to be."

"Not yet, but I'm aiming for about fourth-fifths of the woman I used to be, which I think is a good thing for both of us. Don't you?"

"It's just that you used to be more, more. . ."

"More *what*?"

"More interesting! You used to talk about books you'd read, articles you wanted to share with me, current events. Sometimes, you even talked about the children. Remember them? There are four of them somewhere in this house, probably doing dangerous things with your hand weights. We used to have real conversations about things that mattered. Now all I hear about is about the point value of potatoes, and why we need serotonin, whatever that is, and soy burgers and points of this and points of that. What is the point of any of this?"

I felt my migraine coming back, this time with nuclear warheads attached. "Well! I'm glad to know how you feel about it. I will now refrain from sharing any further nutrition related news bulletins with you. I will make it my day's mission to be interesting for you when you return from work this evening."

"You don't need to be flippant. I think you need to just take a break today. You're getting carried away. Go write an article or something. Don't exercise."

Jeff went off to work, and I tried to fend off my migraine with another cup of coffee. I thought about what he said. Was he right? Had I become a blithering points prattler? Was I really boring him? Was I boring *everybody*? Come to think of it, my friends had been calling less frequently. Even e-mail volume was down.

I thought I'd take his suggestion and avoid The Sculpted Self for the day. Instead, I decided to go to the art museum, where I had wanted to go for the past six years. Somehow, I never found the time.

I bypassed the special visiting exhibit, "Urinals From Uruguay: A Retrospective," and another one called "Bourgeoisie Bites," since all the sculptures were made out of imitation bacon bits and tinned luncheon meats. I had read about that one, since much of it was paid for at taxpayer expense and some people who did not understand modern art were not pleased about it.

I headed straight for my favorite art: anything painted in Europe before 1940. Lo and behold, I was not disappointed. Painting after painting reminded me that in the old days, being a size two was not the gateway to social status that it has become. In fact, based on these paintings, the fashionistas of old were fleshy babes, their limbs draped in shimmering silks. I was happy to see a few Dutch Masters in the museum, although they were tucked way in the back, so as to make room for more modern offerings, such as the one about the urinals. This was giving me a new perspective on things, that's for sure. No matter what the theme, most European painters of more than a century ago usually painted women as at least a size sixteen. Rubens excelled in this, and if he were alive today I would write to him and thank him.

I was particularly struck by a Flemish painting of a naked, smiling courtesan, rosy-cheeked, broad in the beam and double-chinned, but the eager expressions on the faces of the fellows waiting in line to see her proved they considered this an asset. The paintings of men and women who were eating, laughing, and playing the dulcimer also had quaint names that I also liked, such as "A Gentlewoman Slicing Gherkins" or "Festive Picnic With Truffles." The subjects in the paintings looked so happy they probably didn't even realize how deprived they were not to have indoor plumbing, which hadn't been invented yet. Sometimes, paintings only showed the last vestiges of the picnics, such as fruit rinds and duck carcasses. The women, standing to the side of the now-empty tables, wore mischievous looks, and I guessed that some of them had polished off the cakes, too.

In this gallery, there wasn't a skinny Minnie in the bunch. Biblical heroines were buxom, meaty magdalenes. Even nymphs were depicted as D-cuppers, with bulked up thighs. There was no "Still Life With Slim-Fast" anywhere to be found. Any man worth his doublet in those days naturally preferred the heftier women. Pound for pound, they were better bets to survive childbirth and could probably outlast a minor famine. Bigger women were also usually richer, so a little more in the larder gave a gal added social prestige. Of course, there is also the possibility that maybe these girls ate whatever they wanted because they had to appear in public with men who liked to wear too-tight pants, high-heeled boots, and velvet caps with dramatic plumes. Under those circumstances, what motivation would any woman have to watch her figure?

I sat down on a bench and studied the paintings for a long time. I wouldn't necessarily want to go back in time and live without indoor plumbing, even if I could be plump as a dumpling and still draw an admiring crowd. But why did things have to become so extreme? Slowly, my headache took its leave of me, and I made sure to visit another gallery featuring ancient Etruscan pottery. This way, I'd have at least a few interesting things to share with Jeff when he came home in the evening.

April 6

My phone has rarely stopped ringing since I have become involved in the fitness lifestyle. In fact, as my popularity at home has plummeted, it has boomed with health professionals in town. Today was typical. "I wish you will come back to my class," Hypnotica said in her breathless tone. I pictured her wearing a bohemian fringed skirt and long dangling silver earrings. "You have talent. And you are humorous." I thanked her, but told her my dance card was filled for now.

Then the Major called, just a friendly reminder to eat enough protein at regular intervals. Dr. Tostarella, who once called me a "toxic time bomb," sent me a "Wish you were here" postcard also advertising a special sale she was having on something called horny goat weed extract. I was not about to call to find out what that was for! A guy named Hal who sells "Herbs For Life" also pesters me regularly. Hal once left a little paper on my windshield announcing that he was looking for "Twenty-Nine People to Lose Fifteen Pounds! Call Now!" and I was dumb enough to call. Really, I was just curious about why he needed exactly twenty-nine people. Would he have called the whole deal off if he only had twenty-eight people? Once on the phone, Hal tried to keep me in a vice-like conversational grip, mangling the English language as he insisted that I probably had more weight to lose than I thought and the longer I put it off, the harder it would be. When I asked about whether his products contained any of those supercharged herbal compounds that have, in some instances, caused people's hearts to leap right out of their chests, Hal admitted that the teas were in fact "non-decaffeinated." Even Mickey, the manager of Bodies by Barbarella, still dangles new membership offers every few weeks, even though I've said "no" as firmly as I can. Carmen from Weight Watchers e-mails regularly about the importance of not skipping meetings.

All this for a girl who was always, always, the last to get picked for sports teams in school. I can still remember the burning shame of being among the last two kids leaning against the school yard fence, waiting for the team captains to make their agonizing decision: take the kid on crutches, or me. "Oh, all right, I'll take Judy," one of the captains moaned. He was just sore because the kid on crutches got taken first.

April 7

I returned to Mandy's Extreme Cardio-Box class tonight, and even plunked down good American greenbacks for a pair of shiny red boxing gloves in the gym's little shop. Even though it was only my second class, I knew I had made progress. My kicks carried more punch, and my punches, more kick. Once again, I channeled any accumulated aggression and hostility toward my punching bag. Frankly, I would guess almost anybody walking into this class and forced to hear rap "music" ("Ah ain't no cri-mi-NAHL!") would suddenly want to sock something hard. Yet my adrenaline pumped even harder when I thought about a client who stiffed me on an editing job, a recollection that made for a really effective series of upper right hooks. I parlayed another ticket I received near the orthodontist's office into a strong set of rapid-fire jabs. I never thought boxing could be so beneficial for my mental health! When Mandy announced it was time to pick a partner for sparring, I looked at the gal closest to me, a tough-looking young thing sporting a bandana and a nose ring. We nodded almost imperceptibly to one another, just two street fighters with a silent understanding.

Unfortunately, when I removed my sweat-drenched gloves at the end of class, the knuckles on my left hand had swollen up again. I asked Mandy what to do.

She looked at my bruised hand and then at the gloves and asked, "How much did you pay for these? These are cheap. Not nearly enough padding, and they're way too big for you."

When I confessed how much I had spent on them, she advised me to return them and recommended a sporting goods store where I could buy better gloves sized properly for women. At home, feeling energized from my workout, I showed Jeff my bruised left hand. I expected a little sympathy.

"Look at that!" he said. "You're going to damage your wedding ring if you keep boxing with it on. Leave your ring at home next time."

I thanked him for his good advice and went to reacquaint myself with some of the kids, two of whom I heard sniggering about my boxing activities. Before I went to the boys' room, I overheard this:

"Yeah, well, if she's boxing instead of going to Boot Camp, at least now maybe the kids at school will stop saying, 'Your mother wears Army boots.'"

"Great. Now they'll ask when she's going to Vegas for a match with Tyson." They laughed riotously. Here, then, was another benefit to my exercise program: The kids found something to agree on, even if it was at my expense. Still, I couldn't wait to come home next week and demonstrate some of my moves, wearing my new and improved boxing gloves. Then we'll see who's still laughing.

April 8

In an effort to become more interesting to my long-suffering husband, I went to the library today with the goal of reading magazines on various topics. But it was hard to break the habit of first going to the health and diet section, where my court shoes had made a well-worn path in the carpet. I took down a book with the captivating title, *Carbohydrates: Your Road to Certain Death*. I read through about half of it until I felt confident that I got the idea, which was that any carbohydrates other than okra and tomatoes can and will cause heart attacks, marital strife, and termite infestations. As proof, the author cited many studies of lab rats who had been given major doses of cocaine, after which they ate themselves to death. I am not sure what all this had to do with me, but the book helped me come to one firm conclusion: In today's overly permissive society, rats are clearly taking too much cocaine, and they really ought to knock it off.

After I had all the health information I could stomach, I went to the periodicals section, where I boned up on the ongoing crisis in foreign currency and the prospects for a stronger euro. I felt that was enough education for one day.

April 9

I'm seeing all these ads for the "Fat Gobbler," a new "miraculous" pill that promises to keep your body from absorbing the fat in foods. Just pop a "Fat Gobbler" before meals, and presto! Its "magical powers" will bind up the fat, as if it is held hostage, and keep your body from metabolizing and storing it.

I'll admit, I was intrigued. But after looking up articles about the product on an Internet health site, the only thing I felt certain that the Fat Gobbler would gobble was my money. Apparently, the active ingredient in the pill is taken from skeletons of crabs and other crustaceans. Its more common use is to help mop up industrial oil spills. Naturally, enterprising minds leaped to the conclusion that it could probably also prevent fat in foods from landing on the hips. I'm betting that this product was produced by the same visionary business minds who are trying to sell me the "Paunch Patch," which I am supposed to apply to a "discreet" part of my body and rub, to help me feel fuller while eating.

One sad truth I have learned over these months is that there *are* things your body can lose, such as muscle tone and memory cells, but fat is *forever*. I have learned that the body works on a "first hired, last fired" basis when it comes to pockets of adiposity. This means that even if you lose 100 pounds, your body clings tenaciously to every single fat cell you ever had. Only the size of the cells shrinks! Each cell is standing by, all too eager to plump up again at the mere mention of the word "croissant."

Well, I suppose that if we are stuck with each other permanently, I'll just keep trying to shrink those fat cells down to size.

April 10

I received a call from a receptionist at The Sculpted Self informing me that as a new member, I was also entitled to a free session with a personal trainer. When would I like to come in for an appointment? I scheduled my session for the following Tuesday, an hour prior to my Latin Dance class, thinking this was an economical use of time. The receptionist advised me to bring in two liters of water and to stretch out beforehand.

At the appointed hour, I met the trainer, Jack. He was approximately the size of my garage. His corded neck looked like a section of a redwood tree. He invited me into his office and we both sat down. He reminded me of one of those brutes from Muscle Mart, only scarier. Jack wanted to be very clear about his credentials, so I would have full confidence in his qualifications to charge fifty-five bucks an hour for a session with him. First, he pointed to the wall, decorated with the framed cover from a muscle magazine, featuring a well-oiled Goliath in a G-string, posed in profile to accentuate his mutated musculature.

"See that? That's ME!" he boasted.

I looked at the photo, then back at Jack, and saw the uncanny likeness. Although I had just read an article about a cosmetic surgeon who had made a splash in the pectoral implant market, I believed that Jack had come by his biceps, triceps and pectorals honestly. He then pointed to another framed photo, this one of three heavily armed soldiers wading through a swamp, wielding machine guns and deadly expressions. Pointing to the soldier in the middle he said, "That's me, too. Airborne Army Rangers, Panama Canal."

I brightened at the mention of the Army Rangers, which we used to sing about in Boot Camp. I mentioned the Major to Jack, and how he, too, had served our country.

"I know the guy," Jack said dismissively. "He wasn't an Army Ranger. Might've been a SEAL, that's all, but I've seen no documentation. Well, if he says so. . ." Jack shrugged, a motion that, given the bulk and girth of his arms and shoulders, was in itself a dramatic sight to behold.

Jack went on to tell me that many other trainers found him intimidating, though I couldn't imagine why. "I don't care," Jack said. "Most of them don't know what the hell they're doing. All they do is yap at you while YOU do all the work. Know what that's called?"

I did not know, but I knew that Jack would enlighten me.

"That's called being your friend. I don't need to be your friend. I need to be your *trainer.*"

I nodded solemnly. He asked me about my goals, and when I began to say I wanted to shed a few pounds he interrupted. "No! You want to get *fit.*" The muscles in Jack's neck had this way of bulging when he emphasized a point. It was fascinating, in a perverse kind of way.

"My mistake," I said. "Sorry!" I preferred not to argue with guys like Jack. They were so sure of themselves, and so big.

"Now, what did you eat for breakfast today?" Jack had a

paper and pencil ready. I was completely confident about this answer. Even Jack would have to be pleased.

"I had three-quarters of a cup of fat-free cottage cheese, a cut-up mango, and a small low-fat muffin that I baked myself." This was my five-point morning special, and I was quite happy with it.

Jack looked angry. "That's gotta stop."

I couldn't believe it. What could be wrong with fat-free cottage cheese and fruit?

"Too much sugar, and no fat. Mango! Why don't you have an apple instead?"

Muscle mogul or not, I would not continue to just sit there and take this anymore. I gave what I considered a clearly articulated, passionate, yet well-reasoned defense of my breakfast. It was full of protein and calcium, which women needed! The mango fairly exploded with antioxidants, and the sugar was all natural! The muffin had bran, and, well, enough said about that! Best of all, I found it satisfying until lunch.

Jack just shook his head, as if wondering how he would ever find enough time to set everyone right about nutritional and fitness Truth as he saw it. He then leaned forward and said, "Listen, I have a mantra, and I want you to repeat it after me."

I had a well developed wariness of people telling me their mantras, but I knew from Boot Camp that military men had this habit of saying things and then insisting that you say it after them.

"Fat . . ." Jack began.

"Fat . . ." I repeated.

"Is. . ."

"Is . . . "

"My . . ."

"My . . ." I repeated, but the suspense was killing me.

"Friend! Fat is my friend!"

"Friend! Fat is my friend!" I parroted.

At long last, Jack looked satisfied. He then asked me about my workout routine, and I told him that on days when I didn't come to The Sculpted Self, I often did workout videos at home. Stupidly, I expected him to find merit in this practice.

"That's also gotta stop," he growled. I seemed to be annoying him. None of my answers were correct.

Again, I launched a defense, and noted with pride that I had a full set of dumbbells, a weighted body bar, step platform, resistance ring, balance ball, and rubber exercise bands at home. In fact, my entire closet had been overrun by exercise gear. My clothes had been dispossessed and were now lying in a heap in a corner of my bedroom. But Jack insisted that these "workouts," as I called them, were fruitless. "All you're doing is burning calories. You're not building muscle."

What was wrong with burning calories? I thought. This was becoming too tiresome to argue.

"But," he jutted a stubby, steroidal finger at me, "I'm willing to run you through a small, mini-workout right now that will be the type of thing I would do with you to get you in shape. Want to?"

I agreed readily. After all, I was a Boot Camp warrior! And I didn't like his implied insults of the Major. I would do the Major proud. Jack, noting my wedding ring, said, "Only thing is, you won't be able to stand, sit, walk or move tomorrow morning. I don't want your husband coming over here and trying to beat the crap out of me."

I looked at him as he sat there with his massive arms crossed.

"I wouldn't lose any sleep over it if I were you," I said.

Before Jack and I went downstairs, he wanted to measure my body for fat quotient. *Here we go again*, I thought. How many times must I endure this? First I had it done at Flab-No-More! And since then I had it done twice at Boot Camp. I didn't need to test it again just yet. But I didn't want to appear chicken in front of this Brobdingnagian of brawn. He used a different little gadget from either of the others I had seen so far. While I cringed, Jack plucked at me in various and sundry places and then did some calculations. After this exhausting mathematical exercise, he pronounced my body fat to be three percentage points higher than my very first measurement in November, and four points higher than that taken by the Major at the end of Boot Camp. I was incensed.

"That's a lie!" I cried, forgetting momentarily to whom I was speaking.

Jack just stood there, threatening to shake the building simply by stepping from side to side. He looked at me menacingly.

"Are you suggesting that there's something wrong with my instrument?"

"God forbid!" I said, blushing. "But I've had my body fat measured twice before and it's never been this high!"

"My instrument is highly accurate. Theirs' must have been off," Jack said.

I was crushed, and followed Jack downstairs for our workout. I began to wonder, however: Could both of those gadgets have been wrong and only Jack's correct? Or, as I began to suspect, maybe Jack had his rigged to make people think they were fatter than they were! I convinced myself that this was the only possible answer, and I felt more determined than ever to show this prodigious primate what I was made of.

Jack and I both toted along our water bottles as we headed toward the workout area. After all, to be taken seriously as a fitness-conscious individual, you must shlep around vats of water all day, and drink as though you were dying of thirst. Jack clucked that my bottle was too small, and that next time I should bring a jug. Really, it seems as if we are all like babies now, each of us needing our bottles with us whereever we go.

I began by laying down on one of those big exercise balls, trying to keep my head from snapping back off my neck as Jack instructed me to do fifteen sit-ups from my prone position on the ball. Then, Jack demonstrated a style of leg lunges, each of which began by lunging backwards, then kicking up forward. After demonstrating, he faced me and held my hands so I would keep my balance as I did the lunges. Before I began, though,

Jack pointed to his center point of masculinity and issued this warning: "Remember, when you come up for the kicks, watch out for the boys here."

That's all I needed, to accidentally damage Jack's other prized instrument! In fear, my heart reached aerobic proportions before I did my first lunge, which I did with utmost care. While I lunged and kicked, Jack told me this was our "honeymoon," since I only had to do ten lunges on each side today. They were fairly easy. But then I discovered Jack wasn't shooting straight with me. After working my quadriceps on a machine, he spun me around on the floor and ordered me to do another set of lunges, this time fifteen per side. I did so with good cheer and, I thought, rather good form. Best of all, Jack's "boys" remained unharmed. Then it was off to another machine to work the pectorals, and then a set of *twenty* lunges per side. I was tired, but I couldn't stop, since Jack issued an order for me to do fifteen push-ups, toes down, followed by another set of lunges. I had no idea how long this would continue, but I hoped not long, as I was dripping sweat and I feared my heart rate was out of control for a woman my age. Mercifully, Jack said we were done. I quickly calculated that in addition to everything else, I had done sixty lunges per leg!

I wanted to think I had impressed Jack. Since he failed to take the opportunity to compliment me, I brought the matter to his attention. "Not bad, eh?" I asked him, while dabbing my sweaty face with a towel.

"Not bad. For your first time, anyway." Always had the encouraging word, that Jack.

With the session over, and me wondering how I would make my wobbly legs get through Latin Dance, this Titan of triceps ushered me back into his office so I could see how affordable these private sessions would be, provided I signed up for three times a week for six months. Of course, the cost per session went up considerably if I only went once or twice a week, or went for less than six months. However, I had just forked over a goodly sum to join the club, so I told him I'd have to think about it.

Jack said he would give me time to think about it, and would call me by dinnertime. Then I went off to rumba some more calories away in Latin Dance.

April 11

Jack was wrong when he predicted that I would not be able to stand, sit, walk or move the next morning after his workout. I could stand, sit, walk and move, until about two p.m. That's when my shell-shocked muscles emerged from their stupor and realized what had happened to them. Then, they got mad. They let me know just how mad they were by inflicting very serious pain on me, just about every place it was possible to hurt. By dinnertime, even my face hurt from all the fierce grimacing it had to do while the rest of me tried to simply put one foot in front of the other, sit down, get up, or perform any other sophisticated movements. Yeah, sure, I showed Jack what a Boot Camp warrior could do, all right. I would hate for him to ever know just how beaten up I felt!

Even the kids noticed something amiss when I failed to leap into action during dinner (my usual routine) to retrieve second helpings or beverages for some needy individual at the table. Tonight, they had to fend for themselves. About time, too.

"What's wrong, Mom?" asked one son, suddenly recognizing between mouthfuls of food that it was not normal for me to take two minutes to get up from a chair, or to yelp in pain while doing so.

"Oh, nothing, just overdid it a little at the gym," I said. They were already ribbing me enough about my workout schedule – I didn't want to provide any more ammunition. Contemplating my pain, it seemed less and less like a good idea to pay Jack fifty-five bucks an hour to do this to me on a regular basis.

Later that night, I made a slow crawl to bed and had to

move very gingerly to get comfortable. In honor of Vote Lawyers Out of Office Day, I snuggled up with three points worth of peanut butter low-fat frozen yogurt. That was some workout, but not much of a honeymoon.

April 14

According to a report I just read, I now meet the minimum standards of physical fitness for women in the military. Sure, if I had to run through the jungle where the sun don't shine, I'd also do it double-time. Still, this news can't be good for national security. In times of crisis, I'd hate to think that someone like me provides the litmus test for physical fitness in the armed forces. Women in their mid-thirties must be able to do thirty-five sit-ups and fourteen push-ups in two minutes. But heck, now even I can do a lot more than that!

Of course, this is just because the government lowered the standards for women in the military, which is about the dumbest place I can think of to lower standards. Even in Boot Camp the Major expected the same thing from men and women. I may write to the Secretary of Defense about this. Hoo-yah!

April 16

From now on, I vow never to read another article promising to tell me diet 'secrets' of Hollywood stars. The last time I did, my oven blew up. These two facts don't at first appear related, but they are.

I've become a sucker for these kinds of articles, even though none of them have helped me with my weight loss goals. But this article promised to reveal how the celebs keep their gams glamorous, their abs solid as oak. One secret is that it is very handy to have a full-time personal trainer on your payroll, as well as a mobile gym that your trainer can help you cart off to use on location. Tom Cruise swears by this strategy. This way, during breaks on the set, you can do several sets of lunges or a yoga routine under professional supervision.

None of these stars admits to ever eating a whole egg, either. I know this because so many of these Hollywood interviews are conducted in trendy bistros over breakfast, where the reporter dutifully notes what the actors eat. It is always an egg white omelet and herb tea, or something else with fewer than 100 calories. These stars don't seem to have much gastronomic imagination.

Me, I don't buy it. First of all, acting is a physically demanding profession. It takes energy to spend that many hours a day preening in front of the mirror, practicing dramatic expressions or searching intensely for signs of aging. And on the set, stars are often tangled up in demanding love scenes, or storming off the set in a huff. At least that's the scuttlebutt. Don't tell me that you can do all that, or even a set of squats, living on egg whites.

The one thing that sounded promising in the article was a recipe for broiled chicken in a raspberry vinaigrette marinade, apparently, a favorite dish of one female star whose triceps are the envy of Hollywood. I tried to make it at home, which is when disaster struck.

I'm still not sure what went wrong. I had just taken a beautiful apple-banana cake out of the oven, which had been baking at a comfortable cruising altitude of 350 degrees. Then I slipped in two full pans of the marinated chicken, since I planned to serve it to company over the weekend. But somehow, the oven got tripped to the self-clean mode — 550 degrees! When I came to check on the birds about an hour later, smoke was filling the kitchen! I immediately turned off the oven, but couldn't remove the chickens since the oven door locks for safety reasons during self-clean mode. That meant my birds would continue to fry, and our guests would have an even lower calorie lunch than I had planned.

As the smoke got thicker, I got scared and called 911. In a few moments, three huge fire engines were on my block, with about eight firefighters spilling out from the trucks in full battle gear, brandishing hoses. "It's only two pans of chicken!" I said, while showing them in. Still, I was mighty glad to see them. After initially checking out the scene in the kitchen, two of the men ran back to the engine to grab axes, and told me to get the kids out of the house. I had to haul two of them out of the bathtub!

I was sad for my poor kitchen, its white walls getting all sooty, and for what? Another low-calorie chicken recipe! As if the world is somehow lacking in this specimen of cookery advice. As I stood outside with my four kids, including two wearing only towels, I heard the shattering of glass as the firefighters broke down the oven door. Then one of them turned on the biggest fan I ever saw in my entire life to blow the smoke out of the kitchen. Since I knew the house was no longer in danger of blowing up, I couldn't resist sneaking a peek at what these brave men were doing. When I crossed my own front door, the fan blew my skirt up in a most indecorous way. I thought of that famous photo of Marilyn Monroe with her upswept dress. I believe my own image suffered in comparison.

After these brave and wonderful firefighters extinguished my low-calorie chicken, they extracted the two pans, which by then were on exhibit for the entire neighborhood on the front lawn. The bottom pan was nothing but ash and a few bone remnants. It looked as if it had been unearthed and carbon-dated at a million years old. But here's the strange thing. The top pan looked, well, kind of crispy good! Then, to the amazement of the neighbors (but not to his family), my 11-year-old son, who never met a piece of meat he didn't like, grabbed a drumstick and declared, "Not bad at all! A little dry maybe, but delicious!"

I suppose this calamity ought to teach me another secret of the stars: Leave specialty cooking to your own personal chef. It's a lot safer that way.

April 20

It's not a good sign when you show up to an exercise class only to discover the instructor is a guy named Guy decked out in tight black shorts and a feather boa. And let's face it: Anyone who names an exercise class "The Grind" is probably not referring to the cry of an aging clothes dryer coping with too many sneakers thrown in.

I had gone to "The Grind" at my Latin dance teacher's urging. Though she was a little mysterious about the exact nature of the class, I had grown to trust Jennifer not to steer me wrong, and she promised us that it would be an "innovative" and fun way to exercise.

When I first arrived and saw Guy adorned with his feather boa, I naively assumed he made a wrong turn on the way to a party in West Hollywood, where he would undoubtedly pop out of a cake. This is Los Angeles, after all. You have to be prepared to see anything at any time. Still, feeling vaguely uneasy, I uncharacteristically took a place at the back of the studio. Soon, a parade of voguish vamps filled the room, most looking as if they had just come from a casting call for an MTV video. There was only one person noticeably older than me, a granny dressed in regulation exercise shorts and a tank top. She hugged Guy when she came into the room. He gave her ripe, yet firm bottom a squeeze.

"You look *hot* tonight, Valerie," he said to her, and then, turning to stoke up the rest of the crowd, said, "And you're all just going to get *hotter!*" The crowd answered Guy with a volley of appreciative war cries. I hadn't sensed this much excitement since my friend Paula threw a Tupperware party and we all ordered so much she won a $1,500 kitchen cabinet makeover. Guy began to play Rod Stewart's "Tonight's the Night," and cooed, "Let the games begin, ladies and gentlemen!" He flashed us a devilish grin along with a hunk of tanned skin – pretty much the only skin that wasn't already exposed. To be sure, Guy was a fetching piece of eye candy, but as he began to bump and grind to the music, urging us all to follow his lead, I was paralyzed with embarrassment. This wasn't the kind of innovation I had expected! This was. . . stripaerobics!

I had heard about stripaerobics in *People* magazine, but my life usually isn't at all like *People* magazine. The moves Guy was making made even belly dancing look like a Mouseketeers routine in comparison. I shrank back into the corner and did what I remembered of the lindy hop, hoping for invisibility. I knew I should leave, yet I couldn't resist finding out what would happen next.

Guy spotted me hiding and shimmied over. "C'mon honey, there's no place for inhibitions *here!*" He tried to take me by the hand and dance with me, not understanding that if word of this ever got back to the rabbi and the women at the weekly Rabbi's Roundtable, I could never show my face in synagogue again. I wasn't sure what the penalty would be for a married woman dancing with an almost-naked guy wearing a feather boa, but I knew it couldn't be good.

"Uh, no thanks," I said, shrinking back and almost falling into the pile of sticky yoga mats.

"This class isn't for voyeurs," Guy admonished. "Just let yourself go!"

He then strutted away and made a naughty gesture involving his tongue and a finger – a gesture that would have gotten my kids sent away from the dinner table instantly. Then, as if on cue, Granny Valerie leaped forward to dance with Guy, both gyrating their hips. I had to admit I admired a woman who shunned the rocking chair for rock n' roll. To the background music of Joe Cocker's "You Can Leave Your Hat On," Valerie peeled off her tank top and tossed it aside, revealing a Victoria's Secret-type bra underneath. The crowd went wild, applauding and catcalling the sexy septuagenarian. At this point, I knew I had to get out fast. First, some people were throwing me nasty looks, resenting my treating the "Grind" class as a spectator sport. But the final straw was when I saw Valerie tuck her Social Security card into a private area and dare Guy to fish it out. I thought I would faint.

Averting my eyes, I fetched my keys and water bottle and sidled my way out of the studio, where a half-dozen men were watching the action and blocking the door, panting heavily. One guy in a Fed Ex uniform seemed a lot more interested in a pick-up than a delivery. I got out just in time, too, as I heard Guy announce in a throaty voice that it was time for lap dancing and everyone should find a partner.

When I got home, one of the kids said, "Wow, Mom, you must have really had a great workout. Your cheeks are still red!"

They'd never believe the truth, even if I had the nerve to tell them.

April 22

Why am I often hungrier more often now that I have lost weight? I wondered this until yesterday, when I learned that the answer has nothing to do with my stronger muscles needing more fuel. Nope, that would be too logical. It has to do with an irksome little hormone called "ghrelin" that surges in the bloodstreams of people who have lost weight, making them hungry and often sabotaging their weight loss! The only sure way to foil the effects of ghrelin is to have your stomach stapled. So, I suppose I either need to live with the hunger, or gain 100 more pounds so I'll be eligible for stomach stapling. Can't scientists come up with any better solutions than this?

April 23

Ingrid's e-mail today reminded me that I should have finished collecting names and addresses for the Coop reunion invitations. In fact, I probably have my expensive journalism education to thank for having figured out how to track down nearly everyone, including Hartley, Lana, and old blue eyes Gary. Next week I'll send out a "Save the Date!" announcement to everyone in the continental United States. Those abroad will have to suffice with e-mail announcements. The reunion will take place at a palatial home owned by an alumna named Bobbi, who had made a killing as a securities analyst. She had also married well and divorced even better, so she was sitting pretty in Beverly Hills. Bobbi lived with a boyfriend, and in fact, many of the unmarried would be bringing others, significant or otherwise.

Ingrid e-mailed me from some mountainous enclave where she was leading something called a "sweat lodge ceremony." I have no idea what that is, and don't want to know. She sounded increasingly excited about the reunion, and said that since she had just become a "certified breath practitioner," she hoped to offer a breath transformation rebirthing workshop for us during the event itself.

"This will be so cleansing for everybody," Ingrid enthused through cyberspace, "especially since some may still harbor ancient grudges about stuff that happened in college. The rebirthing process will unlock creativity, release inhibitions as well as long-buried childhood traumas!"

Well, maybe. As for me, I'm simply going to arrange to receive an emergency call from the baby-sitter while this is going on. Having been born once and having given birth four times is quite enough birthing experience for me, thank you just the same.

Since she sounded so pleased that I had cut back on my sugar consumption and was exercising regularly, I did not have the heart to confess to her my frequent lapses involving doughnuts. Why dampen the woman's spirits? She also urged me to go try Kundalini yoga, which she said would help me release potential energy and be truer to myself. Frankly, after these months of self-examination, writing down everything I was eating, and allowing all manner of strangers to pinch my fat to test my body composition, I wasn't sure how much more truth I could take. And besides, I had learned that people in this business of health and fitness made an awful lot of sweeping and grandiose promises about various exercise routines. However, it turns out that Ingrid's friend Morrie taught at the Chakra Energy Center, which was in the neighborhood, and she even took the liberty of telling him I'd be coming. I didn't really mind. I was nothing if not bold about trying new things, and after surviving my session with Jack, I thought I could endure just about anything.

At the Chakra Energy Center, I paid for the class, removed my shoes and took a mat, blanket and pillow into a vast, dark room. I had no idea what the blanket and pillow were for, but everyone else took them so I did too. A sign outside the door said we were entering a zone of silence, and people were extremely obedient. And yet, with no apparent sense of embarrassment, people were breathing more vigorously and dramatically than I think is seemly in public. If not for these irritating breathing sounds, I probably would have wanted to curl up on the blanket and pillow and take a nap in this nice dark room. Maybe a nap would help me release my potential energy, a lot of which had been hijacked by my session with Jack.

I put my mat down in the middle of the floor, and was visually accosted by a floor-to-ceiling sized photograph of the Ram Das. His penetrating gaze seemed to convey a knowledge that my preferred method of reaching nirvana, so far, involved military maneuvers or boxing my heart out in a sweaty gym, not lying on a blanket as if I were still in kindergarten, waiting for someone to tell me in a hushed tone to breathe deeply and pose like a cat. I looked away from the photo of the Ram Das, not liking the implication written all over his beard. The enormous platform at the front of the room was piled so high with pillows that for a moment, it almost looked like a gigantic bed. To the right of the platform there were two gongs and a set of bongos. What the heck were we going to do in here? Even though the teacher had not yet appeared, everybody seemed engrossed in something important. A middle-aged woman in front of me rocked to and fro on her feet and flapped her palms back and forth energetically, looking as if she wanted to take flight. Soon, her flapping and rocking grew wild, and she began to hyperventilate. Was she trying to perform an exorcism on herself?

A man placed his mat and blanket down right behind me, in a very orderly fashion, and then stood on his head for a long time. A guy with dreadlocks rubbed oil on his legs. Others were twisting their bodies into inhuman shapes.

About a half hour after class was supposed to have started, a thin man wearing white pants, a long white tunic, a white turban and a gray beard swayed into the room, barefoot. He carried a guitar, which in my opinion was an odd piece of exercise equipment.

I wondered if Ingrid knew that her old friend Morrie had changed his name to the Guru Hari Ram Sada Parwha Singh. Guru Hari darkened the room further and put on a tape of bizarre chants. He then sat down cross-legged and announced that he was devoting this session to transcending space and time, expectations and energy, love, hate, and the mundane. I didn't know what that all meant. I gave him my full attention, but the more he talked, the less I understood. Like the photo of the Ram Das, Guru Hari also seemed to bore through my eyes when he looked at me. Frankly, even though he was a lot less imposing physically, the Guru Hari made me much more nervous than Jack had. Jack just wanted my body, which already made his judgment suspect. But this guy wanted my *soul*. No way would I introduce myself to him later, as Ingrid expected me to. Not only that, I had paid to do yoga, but instead only got a lecture about the contraction and expansion of energy, the big bang theory, the futility of war, the absurdity of futility, and the futility of absurdity. I had never dared take any psychedelic drugs in my youth, but if I had, I would guess that this was what a bad trip might have been like. The Guru Hari also insisted that we must all live the way *we* wanted to live, to be only the people *we* wanted to be! We could not be limited or blocked by external expectations! It was a hosanna to self-absorption.

Listening to the Guru Hari Ram Sada Parwha, formerly Morrie, I wondered: Was this the result of eating tofu in excess over the course of a lifetime? Personally, I wasn't going to chance it. When this insufferable swami pointed his thin finger at us and predicted a day when no false gods would ever darken the doorways of the world again, and instead, we would *all* be gods, a few people on their mats were overcome with emotion, and, despite the vow of silence, broke into whistles and applause.

Mercifully, the Guru Hari finally shut his bearded trap and told us to sit cross-legged and flap our palms back and forth.

"Ong!" Guru Hari began.

"Ong!" The multitudes in spandex and cotton sweats repeated. I thought, I could do this. "Ong" wasn't so hard.

"Ongnamogurudevnamo!" Now Guru Hari and the crowd issued the mantra repeatedly. I, however, was still stuck on "Ong!"

Unfortunately for me, there were only about a half-dozen yoga positions during the entire ordeal, since the Guru Hari had so much to say, and only two hours in which to say it. As the session drew to a close, we had to all lay down on our mats and blankets and close our eyes, as Guru Hari played some more chants. In a moment, the gongs went off. I opened my eyes to peek, and watched Guru Hari gong the concepts of space and time, expectations and energy, love, hate, and the mundane out of us.

When he finished, we were told to open our eyes and sit up. Retrieving his guitar, the Guru Hari strummed serenely on the instrument while the guy with dreadlocks joined him on bongos. They began to sing about love, sunshine, pure light, and other ethereal topics. Everybody except me sang along. I was too busy rolling up my mat and gathering my belongings. I couldn't wait to get home and try to transcend this experience by putting in a Richard Simmons tape. At least that way I'd get some exercise and a couple of laughs, too.

April 26

Yesterday I did the smart thing and popped in another aerobics tape at home. This one devoted a lot of time to weights and to developing my rotator cuff, which I didn't think was really necessary because I could almost swear that we had that replaced when we took the car in for the 60,000 mile maintenance. Obviously, guys like Jack don't want me exercising at home since there's no money in it for them. And another thing I am realizing about a lot of these fitness jocks and diet buttinskys: They all talk a good game about "commitment," but almost none of the ones I have met are married!

I think I now know what Ingrid must have meant by a "sweat lodge ceremony." Clearly, she must have been doing Bikram yoga. I learned about Bikram first-hand today, and cannot understand why it has become so popular. First, Bikram yoga features the most inhuman contortions I have ever seen outside of a freak show, and worse, the exercises are performed in a room where the temperature has been set permanently to "broil." The theory is that all this twisting and sweating helps release your "chakra," or energy. It also mimics the climate of India, when you could toast chapatis on the sidewalk.

Naturally, I have only myself to blame for falling for this. I had foolishly let Ingrid know that my Tuesday with Morrie had been extremely disappointing. She then instant-messaged me to try Bikram instead, pointing out that the international Bikram headquarters just happened to be close to my home. How lucky could I get?

I had become skeptical of Ingrid's advice, so I called in advance to make sure Bikram would provide real exercise and not a lecture on the cosmos. "Don't worry. This is real work," replied the young man at the center, almost sarcastically. I became worried about the cost when I got to the center and saw a sign on the door that said, "Financing available. Easy terms." But even the shock of the cost of a single class paled in comparison to the shock I received when I entered the yoga class itself and discovered that the room was sizzling hotter than a barbecue grill on Labor Day. When my glasses finally unfogged, I realized I was uncomfortably close to a bunch of strange men wearing nothing but Speedos and tattoos, and an equal number of scantily clad women. Monsoons of sweat poured out of them and onto their towels. I found this really distasteful, from an aesthetic standpoint. But ever the naïve fitness wannabe, I was stuck in this carpeted sauna wearing a t-shirt and long exercise pants.

According to Bikram, originator of this discipline, the sweat was a very good thing, detoxifying and all that. And our nose-pierced teacher, Maeve, warned that it was "normal" for new-comers to experience dizziness and nausea sometime during the session, although I had already experienced that when I paid for the class. "Just stick with it," Maeve said about these symptoms. "It will pass." I wondered if this second wave of un-pleasantness would happen before or after I collapsed from heat stroke.

I had done several other yoga classes in the past, and won-dered why so many of the poses expected of human beings were named for non-humans: "cat pose," "table shape," "boat pose," "cobra." But Bikram hadn't raked in enough rupees to drive a Rolls Royce just by offering the old standard "down-ward dog" and "sun salute" poses. No, the sessions he designed entailed twenty-six poses, or "asanas," (a word that sounds sus-piciously close to "asinine"), most of which took the idea of bodily contortions to a whole new level and included one that even Maeve jokingly referred to as "heart attack on a stick." Advanced students could stand on their hands and flip their entire lower bodies behind them, cross-legged. Yet Bikram in-sisted that these poses could cure just about any illness known to man, including diabetes, high blood pressure, emotional un-availability, and excess cash flow.

As I tried valiantly to stand with my legs wide apart while pressing my sweaty face against my feet, I had to face facts: It was time for a pedicure. But as Maeve passed by me, I heard her say,

"Bikram would be very unhappy to see you in this pose without your knees locked." I found this statement vaguely threatening. I feared that Bikram, wherever he was, might channel his multi-million dollar karma and put a curse on my chakra, to punish me for violating the integrity of his tuladandasana position. After all, any guy who had the entire inferno-ized segment of the yoga market all tied up, undoubtedly in the sputa vajrasana pose, was probably a guy with connections. I locked my knees to protect my chakra, and hoped that I would not wreck my spine. If Dr. Charles could have seen me, he would have had a fit! All my other aerobics instructors, as well as the Major, instructed me *never* to lock my knees while exercising.

During the hour-and-a-half class, Maeve issued a rapid-fire volley of instructions that I found hard to follow. "Now sit in lotus position, swing left leg over right knee while right shoulder tilts towards sun, hands in prayer position, inhale deeply, abs tight, shoulders relaxed, mind clear, quickly move into tirkanasana pose. . ." I might have been able to follow these better if I understood Sanskrit and if my brain hadn't been humidified beyond repair.

Another newbie, desperate for air, made the mistake of opening a back door. Maeve skipped over to her and said this was forbidden. The door closed, and the woman passed out. I was too stubborn to allow myself to fail, and I stayed tough. Possibly, I succeeded because I excelled at the "prayer position" and begging for God's mercy in keeping me from falling on my asana. Toward the end, Maeve warned us that it would be normal to have "very strong emotional reactions" to the pose we were doing. She was right. My reaction to being asked to throw my entire body behind my head and rest on the back of my neck — for a full sixty seconds — was simply, "Get me the hell out of here!"

Although I lasted through this trial by fire, I will not return to the Bikram yoga center. It might make me supple and provide me with vibrant good health, but I cannot stand to have sweat in my eyes. Also, at these prices, Bikram would continue to collect Rolls-Royces but I would have to sell my car and live over a street grate. And like they say, if you can't stand the heat, get out of the chakra!

April 29

Someone is going to be in big trouble around here. This is because, despite my having taken extreme precautions with my stash of low-cal treats, my last "Skinny Cow" low-fat ice cream sandwich has been eaten. The perpetrator of this cruel deed may or may not have been the same individual who found and ate my last bag of ninety-four percent fat-free popcorn, my last "Choco-Futti" thirty-calorie frozen pop and, proving that this person must really have been desperate, even my last Weight Watchers two-point bar. I had been cleaned out! *Now* how was I to celebrate the anniversary of the patent for the zipper, awarded in 1913?

My sweet tooth, always on overdrive, was anxious, and I had nothing with which to soothe it. These food filchers could not even begin to appreciate the weeks and months it took for me to discover the existence — and location — of these dieters' delights.

Obviously, only the kids could have been so careless as to have torn into the packages that had the words, "PROPERTY OF MOM: EAT AT YOUR OWN RISK!" written on them in heavy black marker. After all, last I checked, I was the only one around here named "Mom." When I found the ransacked packages dumped carelessly on top of the kitchen garbage, I retrieved them and ran around the house, waving the empties. "Have you no pity?" I asked the children. "After all I do for you, can't you leave my low-calorie things alone? Fess up now! I need names!"

Of course, none of the four suspects of low-fat larceny claimed to know anything about it. I just stood there, with a lean and hungry look, and warned them that dire consequences would result from any further incursions into my treasures. The "Skinny Cow" ice cream sandwiches were a particular loss. Only 130 calories, and two grams of fat for a generous-sized portion! According to the label, even the cows who sacrifice their milk to make the low-fat ice cream for "Skinny Cow" sandwiches are kept on a strict exercise program, followed by regular steam baths and massages. Not a bad life for a cow, if you think about it. In any case, I'm off to the stores now to restock. While I'm out, I'll think of better ways to safeguard my things, such as a chain-link fence around the freezer.

MAY

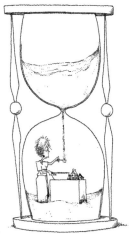

Sweat Gets In My Eyes, But I Also Get New Clothes

May 2 (down eight pounds)

Now I've heard everything. An esteemed national publication has just printed an article that claims that drinking too much water can kill you. The newspaper even ran a photo of an athlete on her way to the emergency room from chugging so much water that she threw off her entire electrolyte balance. One doctor said that in rare cases, too much water can make your cells explode.

This news was inevitable. Eventually, somebody wearing a white lab coat and armed with a federal grant will probably conclude that even broccoli may prove fatal. Stay tuned!

May 5

I saw Marlene at a kid's birthday party where we had both taken our children. She hadn't seen me in several months.

"Wow! You've lost *a lot* of weight!" Marlene said to me.

"Well, a few pounds," I said. I didn't want to exaggerate my unbelievably minor progress. Eight pounds is not that much, after all.

"No, no. It must be about twenty pounds. I can tell!"

Marlene was insistent, and she looked impressed. I told her I only wished it were twenty pounds, but I was haunted for the rest of the day by the nagging question: How must I have appeared to her *before*?

May 6

In honor of No Diet Day, an event that doesn't get nearly the attention it deserves, I conducted my own aerobics class in my closet, where I summoned every ounce of aerobic energy in my possession and threw half my wardrobe into a bag earmarked for charity. I set the radio to a Latin station and rumbaed my way around the closet, enthusiastically tossing my now-too big skirts, dresses and jeans. I danced and tossed vigorously, though I had to be careful not to trip over my dumb bells, Pilates resist-a-ring, yoga mat and other exercise paraphernalia. I cha-chaed my way through the hangers, unearthing the jeans I bought last November. Into the bag they went! Switching to a mambo move and thrusting my hips from side to side for good measure, I yanked a denim skirt off its hanger, one that had been too tight last year, and lassoed the unwanted thing over my head several times before flinging that in, too. I sambaed my heart out, working up an admirable sweat while chucking clothing with abandon and halving my wardrobe in less than an hour.

I considered keeping some things for alterations, but since most of my wardrobe came from places like Target, it hardly seemed worth it. Since I do not know how to sew, it's hard for me to appreciate the very concept of tailoring. Besides, in another few weeks Nordstrom would host their semi-annual women's wear sale. I'd be ready!

Strangely, despite my measly eight-pound drop, I have lost three whole inches from my waist, two from my hips, an indeterminate amount from my upper arms, and three from my hair. I had run to my hairdresser, Lori, for the same cute pixie haircut that Karen Voigt modeled on some of her earlier videos. My physical similarity to Karen probably ends right around the back of our equally shorn necks, but my short locks make me feel young and also keep me a little less sweaty after a good workout.

After I finished paring down my own wardrobe, I got rid of some of Jeff's things, too. I hope he won't notice, but one Hawaiian shirt should be enough for any man. And even though he has maintained the same physique that he had in college, he needn't taunt me by holding onto clothes from that same era. Those clothes already became "retro" and then passé. If he questions me about any of the missing shirts and slacks, I'll just feign ignorance.

When I finished dancing through our closet, I filled another bag with clothes the kids had outgrown. Then I got dressed, jumped in the car with my haul, and deposited the booty at Goodwill, singing all the way. Afterwards I hot-footed it to the mall, where I bought two new skirts in a size I have not worn since I was married! I limited myself to the two skirts, not being really secure about how much more whittling I will manage. Ah, but victory is sweet – even sweeter than a Sara Lee French cheesecake.

May 8

Why is nothing in life simple or straightforward? With spring in full bloom, women's magazines are shouting headlines like these: "Lose Ten Pounds by June!" or "Walk Off Five Pounds in Four Weeks!"

Oh, sure. Easy as pie. Particularly the pies they also want me to make for Mother's Day and graduations. Easy as the basic cookie dough recipe on page 136 that I can easily adapt into fifteen different types of "fabulicious" cookies. So, which is it, editors? Am I supposed to spend my copious spare time exercising and keeping a food diary to get the ten pounds off by June, or exercising my rolling pin until I am roly-poly again? One thing's for sure. They cannot expect me to just bake these pies, brownies and cookies and not double-dip into the batter.

Okay, I can ignore the recipes. But it is harder to ignore the growing chorus of voices trying to deprive me of some of my calorie-challenged snacks.

Yesterday, for example, I arrived at the Rabbi's Roundtable class with an ice-cold can of diet soda. When Tanya saw me, she pursed her lips in disapproval.

"Don't drink that," Tanya said. "That Pseudo-Sweet they use is poison!"

Oh brother, I thought. There's nothing worse than a re-formed something-a-holic. Besides, she could have focused on the positive, such as my new, smaller skirt. But no! She had a one-track mind. My friend Sharon, who, like me, had yet to find salvation in a soy-based life, just rolled her eyes.

"Don't you think that's a little extreme, Tanya?" I asked, deliberately flipping off the top of the can and taking a long, meditative drink. These days, Tanya thought everything caused brain damage, including cooking in Teflon pans. And it had been Tanya to suffer through a nasty cold last winter, while I stayed in the pink.

"No, I don't. The FDA should never have allowed it in foods in the first place. If you look at the studies. . ."

I drank my soda as Tanya delivered a stinging indictment of the offending beverage, which she claimed had a disease-inflicting rap sheet long enough to have shamed John Gotti. I became uneasy. Even though Tanya had become a little hard to manage since declaring her body a white flour- and sugar-free zone six months ago, I had to admit it: She looked incredible.

Her skin glowed. Her eyes shone luminously. When I complimented her on this the week before, she chalked it up to eating a "toxin-free" diet. I suppose she had wheat grass and royal bee jelly flowing through her veins now. On the other hand, it was Tanya, not me, who had gotten sick last winter. In any case, if Tanya were correct about Pseudo-Sweet, it had dire implications for me. Not only would it knock out the no-calorie sodas, which wouldn't be so terrible, but also, more ominously, my thirty-calorie Choco-Futti frozen pops and a few other treats that had only two points or fewer.

And Tanya wasn't the only one on this bandwagon. Last week, I heard it from a hypnotist, and that was even before she led me to a deep theta state of consciousness. I went to Erika Mammon, Ph.D. and hypnotist to the stars, to see if she could help me battle my ongoing sugar cravings. But I became suspicious of her almost immediately.

First, she began by testing me for "suggestibility" — the scientific term for "gullibility." To determine my suggestibility, I had to close my eyes and imagine many strange things. Dr. Mammon asked me to react to the feeling of a helicopter landing on my right shoulder, and then to the sensation of flying in a helium balloon up to the sky. Based on my responses, Dr. Mammon was satisfied that I was indeed "very suggestible" and therefore an excellent candidate for several thousands of dollars of hypnosis.

I was further suspicious of the doctor's multiple treatment plans. For one price, I could learn to love my body "as is," which made it sound like a used car that leaked oil. A higher price would buy me enough hypnosis to help me pare myself down to a svelte size four. Dr. Mammon didn't realize that no female ancestors in my direct bloodline had ever been a size four. A thorough genealogical study of my family proved that all my female forebears carried the same dominant "Z" gene ("Z" for zaftig) that kept us in a perpetually pleasingly plump condition. Aspiring to become a size four seemed not only undoable but also too shallow a goal, even for me. Then, as a casual aside, Dr.

Mammon said, "I hope you aren't drinking diet sodas." She looked at me expectantly as she said this, her expression a severe warning.

"Well, actually, I have two or three a week," I said.

"That stuff destroys brain cells!" Dr. Mammon nearly shrieked.

"Really? How do you know?"

"I used to drink a six-pack of diet soda *every day*, for almost *thirty years!*"

I wondered if Dr. Mammon understood the implications of her confession. I wondered which was more deleterious to one's brain capacity: drinking a few diet sodas made with minuscule amounts of Pseudo-Sweet each week, or agreeing to fork over thousands of dollars for the privilege of wearing funny sunglasses with flashing red strobe lights over your eyes and being asked to bark like a dog.

Still, Dr. Mammon obviously had many functioning brain cells, since she sure knew how to fill that waiting room of hers with oodles of suggestible patients. They must have made it much easier for her to make payments on that shiny new BMW in the parking lot.

I'm still spooked enough to not buy any more of my Pseudo-Sweet treats, even the thirty-calorie Choco-Futti pops. But how unfair! Not only am I supposed to give up refined sugar, but also its substitute! Under the circumstances, I had to commemorate Sonny Liston's birthday with a nectarine.

My universe of sweets is shrinking a lot faster than I am.

May 10 (51 days before Coop reunion)

With the Coop reunion less than two months away, it's pretty clear that I will not achieve my original goal of dropping fifteen pounds for the occasion – unless they postpone it for another year. But I am trying not to worry about it, especially since I am so happy to be a size smaller. Anyway, I have a new, more urgent goal now, which is not to allow exercise to make me into a total cripple.

This became clear to me today, when my chiropractor, Dr. Charles, reviewed recent x-rays of my spine with me. These scary pictures revealed that my spine, crooked since birth, is now buckling like the interstate highway after a massive earthquake. And since I've been exercising so regularly, my lower back has been stiffer and achier than usual. Dr. Charles didn't blame this on exercise alone; the aging process is taking care of a lot of that without any outside assistance. And if I were not exercising, I'd be even worse off.

I looked at my x-rays on the screen, where my spine assumed the ghastly likeness of a cobra. That just figured! Here I was, trying to help my wonky spine, but some activities, I now realize, are just rushing me headlong (and spine-long) toward gimphood.

Dr. Charles assured me that as long as I avoided running, jumping jacks, and other high-impact exercises, I would probably not end up needing handicap access to public places. He offered this reassurance after we finished looking at the depressing pictures and while ushering me to the torture chamber called the "distraction-flexion" table. I just call this two-pronged table "the rack," since it reminds me of something they might have used during the Spanish Inquisition. Dr. Charles puts me on the rack every once in a while to keep my vertebrae from going into total lock-down position. While I lay face down, I took the opportunity to complain into the table's small breathing space about the unfairness of my having worked so hard for a less than ten-pound loss. I yammered on as he tied the leather straps around my ankles and pulled them tight. While I held on for dear life to the hand grips above my head, Dr. Charles began to swivel the bottom half of the rack hither and yon. This scares me because Dr. Charles twists many things that I use on a daily basis, including my entire lower spinal column.

"If you had had fifty pounds to lose instead of just fifteen, you would have lost a lot more. Don't worry about the pounds," he said, while cranking my nether regions around as if I were a ball bearing. *Swivel, twist, wamble!*

I know that Dr. Charles only inflicts this pain on me with the best of intentions. Still, being on the rack is even scarier than when he takes my head in his two hands, rolls it around a little, then instructs me to "relax" before yanking my neck from side to side. We know this maneuver has worked if we both hear that satisfying "snap, crackle, pop" sound of my ligaments being forcibly rearranged. I have always wondered how the heck these doctors have the nerve to tell you to "relax" when they have strapped you down on a table, or, in the case of the ob-gyn, have your feet in stirrups while zeroing in on your most private area with a cold, shiny steel implement. Do they have theatrical training?

Looking at the bright side, I never liked jumping jacks anyway.

May 12

After surviving three family celebrations in the past two months cake- and ice cream-free, today I broke down for my youngest son's tenth birthday. I had gone an unbelievable 162 days without so much as a lick! But even tonight, I only had about four spoonfuls. Five, tops.

This has taught me that when the pressure is on, I can live without ice cream. But I cannot live without chocolate.

The proof is that I went to a Chocoholics Anonymous meeting to try to kick the habit. I don't know what possessed me exactly, other than that I was overly confident last week after the Great Closet Cha-Cha and Garage Sale. I figured, it really hadn't been that hard to cut back on the fats, the carbs, the ice cream. But could I go cold turkey on chocolate, my gastro-nomic passion? Certainly, if I dropped chocolate as one of my four major food groups I would stand more of a chance of shak-ing off those last pesky pounds. I might even become a person of greater character. At least, that was the theory. But I knew I couldn't do it alone.

I had never been to a twelve-step program before, and clearly had no idea what I was getting myself into. When I arrived at the meeting, the leader, Thomas, read the group's credo:

"We, the members of Chocoholics Anonymous, are a fellowship of men and women who have admitted our powerlessness against chocolate, whether milk chocolate or bittersweet, with or without nuts or nougat. We believe in freedom through total abstinence of chocolate, and have given over our dependency to God, whom we believe only created chocolate by accident. He Himself never touches the stuff."

After this introduction, Thomas invited newcomers to introduce themselves. A woman raised her hand, and rose from her seat.

"Hi. My name is Geraldine, and I'm a compulsive chocoholic."

The entire room, except for me, who didn't know I was supposed to do this, all shouted, "Welcome, Geraldine, compulsive chocoholic!" They looked at her, expecting her to say something more. She didn't disappoint them.

"This group has meant so much to me since I joined last Thursday. My sponsor has checked in with me three times a day, and once she got me just in the nick of time, as I was on the verge of ripping open a Mars bar."

Every face in the room radiated sympathy. Several heads were nodding slowly.

"I've had other addictions before," Geraldine went on. "Soap operas. Computer backgammon. Department store gift-with-purchase cosmetics sales. But nothing has threatened my stability as much as my chocolate addiction." Oh sure, it had all started innocently, with a slice of fudge birthday cake when she was three years old. But over the years, Geraldine's passion for chocolate simply got out of hand. All pretense of self-control melted like so many M&Ms under the hot summer sun. Geraldine then told us what finally drove her to seek help:

"When my boss caught me with my hand in his candy jar, scooping up some York peppermint patties, I was filled with shame. He questioned my loyalty to the company. 'What kind of individual would stoop so low as to steal somebody else's York peppermint patties?' he asked. I knew that my credibility in other areas was also on the line. That's when I came here."

She sat down, wiping away tears. Thomas thanked her for her brutal honesty. "Any other newcomers today?" Thomas asked, looking straight at me. I felt trapped. My heart pounding, I, too, rose.

"Hi. My name is Judy, and I'm a compulsive chocoholic." I didn't like the sound of the word "compulsive" coming out of my mouth.

"Welcome, Judy, compulsive chocoholic!" After this cheery greeting, everyone waited for me to spill the beans. Who did these people think they were, anyway, expecting me to disclose some of my most private secrets? They were total strangers. This was none of their business. But I had to say something.

"I was born in a little log cabin in the mountains, where we lived a simple life," I began. Looking around, I saw that some people looked perplexed, perhaps because I didn't have a log cabin accent. I decided to try one on for size.

"But when my Daddy had the chance to move us to the city and get a job in the foundry, all kinds of new opportunities opened up for us. Indoor plumbing. Book learnin' in school. Big city supermarkets with aisles full of candy. *Chocolate* candy." Surveying my audience, I could see I had them now. One woman slid all the way to the edge of her seat. They were like putty in my hands.

"Go on," Thomas prodded gently. "You're safe here. Nothing you say will ever leave this room."

For the next twenty minutes, I had them spellbound by my chocolate addiction, a fantastic tale of depravity that began with my maiden cup of hot chocolate in kindergarten, and progressed over the years to a wild compulsion that eventually got me in trouble with the law. It started small: pilfering some Reese's pieces packages or cold cartons of chocolate milk. But before long I was hooked on the hard stuff: Häagen-Dazs. Godiva. Belgium chocolates I got on the black market. After I was released from juvenile hall, where the desserts were pretty awful, I got a job in a bakery, but I always ate all of my salary, and then some.

Soon, friends stopped trusting me in their pantries. Relatives feared that I would show up at family functions wearing an embarrassing chocolate mustache and get chocolate stains on the good tablecloths. Everyone feared my bad influence on children. I finally bottomed out in a cheap motel room, where the police found me slumped in front of the television, where an infomercial described the fantastic results of a revolutionary do-it-yourself laser surgery kit. I was in a full-blown ice-cream-induced brain freeze, mumbling the words "Chunky Monkey" over and over again. The dingy room was strewn with empty boxes of Russell Stover chocolates, See's Candies, and Hershey wrappers. On my unmade bed was the book, *Death by Chocolate,* open to a page containing a recipe for something called "Fatal Fudge Bars." My family scraped enough money together to put me in detox so I could dry out for a few days. After that, they said, I was on my own. This brought me to Chocoholics Anonymous, where I hoped to stay clean.

I finished my story and wanted to sit down, but the crowd stampeded toward me as if they were bulls in Pamploma, just let out of the pens. All they wanted was to give me a group hug, but I hate group hugs. The woman who had been on the edge of her seat got to me first and sobbed on my shoulder. Others followed suit. After this great emoting of the gathered chocoholics, I managed to peel the rest of them off of me and sit down. I felt like a cad. It got worse when people began vying to become my sponsor. People began shouting at one another. Things got ugly. As group leader, Thomas then made an executive decision that he would sponsor me, just to end the squabbling.

By the time I got home from the meeting, Thomas had already called me twice on my cell phone, to make sure I hadn't made any unauthorized stops at a 7-Eleven. When he heard the exasperation in my voice during the second call, he explained the importance of my having enough support, particularly given my history. Still, Thomas' calls annoyed me. And I began to fear that someone might discover that my story lacked a certain verisimilitude. In my defense, I did try to stay chocolate-free. I lasted a full thirty-six hours, but Thomas' incessant phone calls finally drove me straight to a bag of Chips Ahoy, where I had two small cookies, which I duly recorded in my Weight Watchers journal.

Whenever I think about all those people spending three hours a week at Chocoholics Anonymous meetings (not including travel time), I shake my head with pity. If they were working out at the gym instead, they could be earning their way to a good-sized chocolate eclair. My experience with this group simply confirms the wisdom printed on my favorite refrigerator magnet. It says, "I'd give up chocolate, but I'm no quitter."

May 14

The worst part about having gone to the Chocoholics Anonymous meeting has been trying to shake this guy Thomas off my tail. He calls all the time. What a pest! I may have to get an unlisted phone number.

May 18

Yesterday I fell back into an old eating habit, but I paid dearly for this lapse in dietary discretion. Too tired to go to the gym, I snuck out to a matinee and got a bag of popcorn and a diet soda. I enjoyed the movie, but my insides absolutely mutinied against the popcorn, now considered by my body an alien and hostile substance. Even in the privacy of these pages I will not describe just how angry my body was with me, but suffice it to say, it taught me a lesson I shall not soon forget. Clearly, I have a new, extremely more sensitized system now, and it expects better than to have a tub full of hydrogenated soybean oil poured down it.

Yet my punishment was not complete until today, when I made the mistake of trying a workout called "Tantric Toning," which promised a sensual workout combining the best of yoga, tai chi, Chi Kung, and, for all I know, Egg Foo Yung. When I popped the video in at home, I saw half a dozen tantrically fit women standing against a backdrop of billowing leopard-themed draperies as an indefensibly beautiful teacher named Zenyth started talking about the earth's energy. She promised to teach us to "be ourselves, naturally!" and to "gather our passionate potential!"

I had a hunch that even Zenyth was not entirely herself, "naturally," and had gathered some of her own potential at a cosmetic surgeon's office. After all, she was the only one wearing a push-up bra, whose copious contents seemed suspiciously out of proportion to the rest of her boyish figure. Zenyth spoke breathlessly, but that may not have been her fault. After all, adding that pair of cha-chas must have taxed her poor little lungs beyond the call of duty.

She talked a good game about working up a fire in the hips and reminded me a little of the belly dancer Hypnotica. But for someone who kept talking about being "at one with the earth," I found her phony, siliconed stockade more than a little distracting.

Zenyth ended the workout with a "color meditation," to infuse our internal organs with dignity or oneness or something like that. I played along for a while, imagining ruby red radiating through my heart to expand my capacity for love and passion. I figured, maybe it would inspire me to go out and buy some nightwear more sensual than a husky-sized Lakers t-shirt one of the kids had won at a birthday party. But by the time we were supposed to let go of our anger by imagining green swishing through our liver, I was through.

Maybe if Zenyth hadn't kept telling me how much I should love myself (apparently, no one but me could manage a job that big), I might not have felt a passion to feel at one with a double-mushroom burger and fries. But the "new me" did not succumb to mere sensuality! I now loved myself enough to push away those naughty ideas, and memories of the popcorn debacle were still painfully fresh. Instead, I ate some leftover lentil soup and a salmon patty for lunch.

The power and pride that tantric toning was supposed to give me only kicked in after I disgorged the tape from the VCR and returned it to the library. I do hope that this exercise tape will one day find its own rightful place at one with the earth – deep, deep, down in the earth, rooted so completely that the rest of the unsuspecting exercising public could feel truly "free" from this video frame-up.

May 20

Here are some of my conclusions after five months of semi-dedicated dieting, energetic exercising and rigorous research:

1. Being overweight is a bad thing. Being over-weighed isn't a whole lot better.
2. Publishers should run criminal background checks on anyone proposing to write a diet book. To me, these authors seem a shady lot.
3. It *is* possible to eat too many "zero-point" vegetables, especially cauliflower and green peppers. They invite heartburn and other unpleasantness.
4. People should have the courtesy to turn off their cell phones during yoga class, particularly if they have set their ringer to play the theme song of "Hawaii Five-0" or "Here Comes the Bride."

5. Joining the words "Lose Weight, Effortlessly!" in the same sentence may be a form of hate speech.
6. Weight Watchers is a very effective and sensible pro gram, particularly if you follow it.
7. Eating a bagel once or twice a week should not induce deep angst in anyone.
8. It is unfair for restaurants to charge more for an egg white omelet than for a regular omelet. After all, they get to keep half the egg.
9. As best as I can tell, "Pilates" (pronounced "Pi-*lah*-tees") is French for "death by leg lift." If only they had in vented this floor routine during the French Revolu tion, there would have been no need for the guillotine. Traitors to the crown could just as easily have been sentenced to twenty years of hard labor with a re sist-a-band and a floor mat. The monarchy would have been safe.
10. Fitness experts are correct that variety is essential in exercise. If I do aerobics on a Thursday, for example, I'll try to do resistance training on Friday. It keeps things interesting and keeps your muscles working. I also ad vise naps on Saturday.
11. There really is no such thing as "spot reducing," unless you have a really good dry cleaner.
12. Being strong and fit feels great, and that can still hap pen if your weight exceeds what the government ex perts claim it should. After all, how often is the govern ment right about anything?

May 22

After a prolonged absence, I returned to Weight Watchers this morning, and was miffed to discover that my registration card had vanished! I marched right over to Carmen to inquire.

"If it's not there, you must have missed more than four

meetings. That means you've been dropped from the program, and you'll have to rejoin. Like I told you before, Weight Watchers is a *commitment.*"

Well, I'd been tossed out of better joints than this! Feeling stung, I realized I was still holding on to a half-dozen boxes of chocolate mint two-point bars for which I was prepared to offer hard currency. I had something in common with my favorite flavor of two-point bar, though. We had both been dumped by Weight Watchers! Last March, they discontinued the flavor, and now in May, they discontinued me! But just as the corporation couldn't keep a good flavor down (mint-loving members stormed the corporate office with protests, forcing an end to the exile and proving that the democratic spirit is still alive and well in this country), I vowed that they wouldn't keep me down, either.

For a few moments, I considered whether I should ante up again for new membership, or simply pay for my bars and go home. While I pondered my fate, I noticed that many of the stalwart members whom I had seen over the past months looked slimmer and slimmer. I had been exercising religiously, but based on my "Thinner" scale at home, hadn't dropped more than another pound since I'd last been there.

So, I did what any other self-respecting woman would do in my situation. I paid for my bars and then threw myself on Carmen's mercy. I reminded her that it was only five weeks since my last attendance and begged her to take me back without paying a penalty. I gave her my most imploring, pathetic look, one that I had polished over many years of practice and applied successfully in many other tight situations. I also showed her my receipt for my armload of two-point bars. Apparently, I hadn't lost my touch. Carmen thawed enough to instruct the busy cashiers, who were no doubt working up a good case of repetitive stress syndrome by swiping through credit cards by the hundreds, to re-register me and charge me only for the meeting and weigh-in.

Still, my old card, with its vital statistics, had been expunged from the record, like a piece of damning history wiped from the books of a repressive regime. I began anew, and dutifully weighed in at a pound lower than I had five weeks earlier.

Carmen's topic of discussion today zeroed in on commitment, and how the lack thereof spelled disaster. She promised that anyone who dropped out now, thinking they could just follow the Weight Watchers guidelines on their own, were living in a fool's paradise.

"I've seen it over and over again," Carmen warned. "You know what happens to people who think they don't need this support and these weekly weigh-ins?"

The crowd was hushed in anticipation.

"They gain back all their lost weight and *more*! Come January, they slink back here like prodigal sons and daughters, filled with remorse! And for what? Avoid this heartache! Just keep on coming, keep on journaling, keep counting your points, and you *will* achieve your goal!"

During Carmen's stirring soliloquy, I thought I heard the strains of "Battle Hymn of the Republic." But then again, it could have been my imagination.

Carmen also dangled the tantalizing possibility that once we reached and then maintained our goal weight for six weeks, we would be eligible for lifetime membership. This was not an offer to be taken lightly. As "lifers," we were entitled to many special privileges, including Lifetime Membership recognition awards and employment opportunities!

When Carmen opened up the discussion, a young lady eagerly raised her hand. I assume she felt somewhat insecure, since she phrased everything – even statements of fact — as questions.

"I ate lunch this week with a skinny person?" she began, "And you know, like, I saw how she ate? I realized that I had already finished my whole meal while she was still, like, tucking her napkin in her lap?"

Carmen leaned toward her audience and pointed at the

speaker. "Take note of this astute observation, ladies and gentlemen! Thin people eat very slowly, while heavy people too often just snarf their meals! Listen, our brains need *twenty minutes* to register that we have food in our systems. Let's remember that and take a lesson from our naturally thin friends. No one's going to take your fork from you, so give it a rest in between bites. Great point. Thank you."

Now that I was again a member in good standing, I felt obligated to add my own observation about thin people. I raised my hand, and Carmen called on me.

"I agree that thin people do eat agonizingly slowly, but I have also noticed that if you hang around a bakery or donut shop, thin people who stop by are only buying coffee, or a single donut for their kid. They, personally, do not eat them."

I saw that some people were looking at me strangely. Carmen said, "I suppose I shouldn't ask what you are doing hanging around bakeries and donut shops. That's a good way to derail your weight loss efforts. Point taken, though. Look, just like that old saying that the rich are different from the rest of us, so are thin people. Unless, that is, we make their habits our own!"

And with that, the meeting ended, and I took my new cache of chocolate mint two-point bars and went home.

May 26

This morning when I went into the kitchen I saw that sometime during the night, we had an impromptu visit by two ants, accompanied by 45,000 of their closest friends. Apparently, they are not the only disgusting creatures in town under the mistaken impression that I am holding a no-host bar event for insects, because termites have also been busily chomping up hunks of the house. Next week, the insects will have the place to themselves, since we will have to move out while the house is fumigated. It seems that almost everything in the house has gone on strike, except for the ants and termites. The dishwasher has suffered some kind of stroke, the front door has frozen itself shut and cannot be opened, and the freezer is making threatening, weird noises. Just when I thought things couldn't get worse, some idiot stepped on my glasses at the gym. I always take them off during sit-ups, and was afraid that someday this might happen. However, I never imagined that the idiot would be me.

I can hardly wait to get on my gloves and hit the bags in Extreme Cardio-Boxing tonight – I've got a lot of hostility to get out of my system.

May 30

I am usually so rushed when coming and going from the gym that I never have time to try the machines. But today I had the luxury of an extra half-hour after yoga class, so I tried to figure out how some of them worked. I couldn't believe how many different contraptions there are for every conceivable muscle group! Although each machine has a diagram and instructions, I still felt befuddled by the equipment. I first attempted a bicep curl machine, mostly because it promised to train my lower trapezius, which I hadn't seen since I was a kid visiting the circus, along with my brachioradalis, which sounded like something extinct.

While I sat on the chair and adjusted the amount of weight, I spied Jack wandering the room, no doubt prospecting for gold. I often saw him prowling around, sometimes supervising his own students, and other times, just looking intimidating. He began lumbering over my way. The guy still made me nervous.

"You're not using this machine correctly." Jack never was one to mince words.

"Really? I tried to follow the diagram," I said, hating to look stupid in front of him.

"You're doing it backwards. You need to pull the weights up, not back. This isn't a tricep machine." Jack's bulk hovered over me like a storm cloud as he demonstrated the correct way to position my arms.

"Thanks a lot, Jack. I really appreciate it, especially since I never signed up for your sessions and all."

Jack squinted in a classic Clint Eastwood expression. "That's just the kind of guy I am," he said.

"Well, you're a real sport, and I appreciate it," I said, now hoisting the weights, which I had set at fifty pounds, in the forward position that he had shown me.

"That's kind of a lot of weight on a bicep curl for a gal like you, isn't it?" he asked.

"I don't think so, Jack," I said, wishing I had set the bar at sixty pounds. I couldn't have kept it up for long at sixty, but I liked the feeling of impressing this Colossus. "As you recall, I am a Boot Camp warrior. But I appreciate your concern."

Jack then swaggered across the room, all 265 pounds of him, only four percent of which was body fat. He returned to the hunt.

JUNE

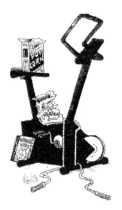

Stand and Deliver

June 3

Supporting an exercise habit requires a steady cash flow. For example, now that I am stronger, I need to buy new, heavier hand weights. Ditto for my old weighted body bar, which at twelve pounds no longer challenges my bigger, buff muscles. The add-on weights that make the bar heavier don't fit *my* bar, whose style was discontinued last year! If I want to continue using this nifty device, I'll have to pony up for a new body bar, in addition to the add-on weights. They get you coming and going in this business.

I suppose I shouldn't complain that I have also exercised my workout clothes into a state of untenable rattiness. And I have only myself to blame for having to buy new glasses. But my biggest upcoming fitness-related expense, other than the tummy tuck still under consideration, will be to replace the floorboards under the carpet in my bedroom. My manic workouts have loosened them, and they now creak madly each time I lunge or leap during an aerobics tape.

And while I'm on the subject of spending money to improve my health, yesterday I finally braved a trip into Shoe Stadium for a new set of sneakers. I felt dizzy just looking at the store's 4,000 different styles of footwear, each of which, naturally, is designed for a different activity. When I flagged down a sales clerk and told her I just wanted a basic all-purpose athletic shoe, she looked at me as if I had fallen from the turnip truck.

"Shoes just aren't that simple anymore," she said. "For example, will your main purpose be for leisure walking, fitness walking, performance walking, or hiking? Do you need lateral cross-trainers or straight-up cross trainers? Will you use them primarily for jogging, basketball, or kick-boxing? It's unreasonable to expect one shoe to do it all."

Yet I held firm, thinking about the new street clothing that I also needed to replace my assortment of too-big clothes. I insisted that four pair of shoes were not in the budget, and asked for her best advice if I were only to buy one pair. She then offered this cryptic advice: "If you insist on only one shoe, you should buy something with an internal engineered arch support, multi-directional performance air pockets, dual-density compression molded EVA, and a molded heel counter for maximum support. Multi-directional outsoles with a lug configuration and lateral outriggers would be helpful."

Huh? Had she really thought this was helpful, or was she intentionally inflicting punishment because she didn't like me? "I'm not sure I follow you," I confessed.

"Look," she said, sighing irritably, "try to find a lateral cross-trainer with a lined insole board and an injected TPU detachable plate. Also, I can see from looking at the soles of the shoes that you're wearing today that you have a problem with underpronation, so I would also suggest something with a firm medial post."

After she walked away, I chose a style all by myself called the "Daisy Cutter." I have no idea if my Daisy Cutters have air pockets or EVA or TPU or EPA or anything like that, but they feel good; I liked the military sound of it, as well as the color scheme (blue with lavender edging). Plus, they were on sale.

I have been called a lot of things in my day, but I have

never been accused of "underpronating," which to me sounds like some kind of crime against grammar and therefore a slur against my professionalism. I can't imagine a new pair of shoes will help much with that.

June 7

The reunion is only three weeks away, and I just ordered my outfit for the occasion. Typically, Ingrid had insisted on stating "casual dress" on the invitations, and I don't want to stand out by showing up in an overtly *haute coutre* ensemble. Therefore, I'm going for a look that says elegant, yet not faddish. Swank, yet not voguish. Casual, yet deadly serious.

I lucked out shopping online with one of my favorite clothing catalogs. Their company offers a "virtual model" so that I will know how their clothing will look on someone unfortunate enough to have my build. After logging on, I customized my virtual model to match my height, weight, proportions (such as they are), hairstyle and facial features. Fortified with this information, and without even being asked, a screen popped up with tips for me to dress with maximum style and minimum embarrassment. The box on the screen issued the following recommendations: "Avoid large motif prints, especially anything with a safari or boating theme. Thick fabrics are not your friend. At all costs avoid mandarin collars and chunky jewelry. To create an illusion of height, wear tights and shoes of the same color. To create an illusion of a bust, select sweaters with bright, contrasting colors. Click HERE for our selection of support undergarments and padded bras."

Keeping this wisdom in mind, I then had my virtual model try on several outfits that I liked, none of which had safari motifs or mandarin collars. Unfortunately, I thought she looked a little dumpy in the dress I liked best, so I went back and customized her to lose five pounds. While I was at it, I changed her hairstyle, and gave her quick reconstructive surgery to accentuate her cheekbones. Boy, this was the easiest makeover anyone ever had! With a few mouse clicks, my virtual model was sheared of excess poundage and smartly turned out. Since she looked so much better now, I ordered the dress in the size that matched her new and improved weight.

It better fit me as well as it fits her by the reunion.

June 12

My weight has been stuck for several weeks now. In the weight-loss industrial complex, they call this situation a "plateau." Stubborn as a teenager, the scale has refused to budge, even though I am exercising five times a week and eating extremely carefully.

In other words, I am friggin' mad.

I complained to Ingrid about this during our last conversation. As always, she had an answer. "I'm sure that the stress of worrying about getting down to your goal weight before the reunion is the only thing keeping the weight on. If you could just grow to accept yourself as you are, I bet that weight would just fall right off."

"Ingrid, weight has never just 'fallen off' me. It isn't like a pyramid of fruit at the market where if you pull one from the bottom, the rest tumble down after it. My fat has been soldered on permanently. I also suspect it suffers from deep-seated attachment issues. For me to lose a pound, I have to machete it off through grueling and inhumane bouts of exercise and an eating regimen that would barely keep a canary alive."

"I thought you liked exercise!" Ingrid asked.

"I do. I even love it! Still, where is my payoff?"

"Your payoff is that you've lost eight pounds and a dress size. You look better and you feel great. Can't you be happy with that?"

"No."

"Okay then. Why not go get a good massage with some

peppermint aromatherapy. At least it will relax you. Maybe, if you want, a high colonic as well. It never hurts to detoxify."

"What's a high colonic? It sounds alcoholic."

Ingrid laughed indulgently. "No, it's nothing like that. In fact, just the opposite." Then, to my horror, Ingrid explained what a colonic really was: a hosing down of my entire upper intestine, to flush out all the built-up toxins and other nasty things that were no doubt nesting in there. Just like with so many other tricks in the holistic health universe, adherents made fantastic claims about the potential of colonics. It would help with everything from carpal tunnel syndrome to psoriasis, insomnia to ingrown toenails. And of course, it would help those trapped, as I am, in a "weight-loss plateau." Having a colonic sounded very similar to having the car radiator flushed, only less dignified. Naturally, for the procedure to be of any value, I should have at least three sessions. But it would all be worth it, Ingrid explained, because as everyone knows, all death processes begin in the colon.

As Ingrid has her pulse on the entire health community, she referred me to Hermoine Strump, a "colonic emancipator and reflexology master." Before I called Strump's office, I looked up colonics in the phone book and was surprised to see how many people there actually were who siphoned off bowel sediment for a living. "Colonic Irrigation" was located just where I expected to find it: after "Collection Agencies" and before "Comic Books." Strump's ad boasted that her colonic procedures were both "safe" and "private." As opposed to what? Unsafe colonics performed before a live studio audience?

I knew that most medical doctors felt that colonics were just tomfoolery, but of course veterans of the embarrassing practice insisted it was a great tonic for health. I debated whether to allow this plunging of my innards as a last-ditch effort to peel off a quick few pounds. I did have other options. But I could not imagine fasting for three days on a solution of filtered water seasoned with lime juice, a teaspoon of maple syrup and cayenne pepper. I did not see the wisdom in spending nearly a hundred bucks on an herbal wrap to make me sweat, when I could just go to the gym and take three consecutive aerobics classes. I was too scared to tank up on Hyper-Meta-Phedra-Bolic, which would speed up my metabolism, but also, perhaps, induce heart failure. I even flirted with the nutty notion of living for a few days on low-cal meal replacements and herbal supplements, until I read a newspaper report about some European women who had lost more then just weight doing this routine – they developed a condition with a long Latin name that caused them to lose muscle coordination and balance. Finally, one gal I met in Latin dance swore by coffee enemas, but I was too shocked by this idea to ask the questions that immediately surged in my brain: Columbian or French Roast? Regular or decaf? Besides, I'm not sure I trust the judgment of a woman who wears thong underwear. I wish she had never mentioned the hideous thing to me, since I could only drink tea for several days afterwards.

I concluded that even though a colonic "emancipation" would involve the hated, dreaded speculum, it still sounded better than these other options. I threw caution to the wind and called Hermoine Strump.

June 14

When it was all over, Hermoine Strump asked me in a hopeful tone if I felt lighter.

"Sure, sixty-five bucks lighter," I said, trying to sound more spirited than I felt after having had what seemed like several hundred gallons of water coerced through my gut. When I first arrived at her office, I smelled burning incense – always a reassuring sign that you are with a real medical professional. But as I climbed on the table, I just about lost my nerve. I tried to work up the courage to ask for a reflexology foot massage instead, but Strump was too fast for me, quickly launching into a sermon about the new universe of health that could open up to me once she irrigated my bowel.

"You won't be sorry," she said as she slipped on her gloves.

I'm sorry already, I thought.

A few minutes later, when I was deeply, deeply sorry, Strump chirped happily as she showed me all the toxic sludge shooting out of my traumatized body. I lay there, hoping that Hermoine Strump, colon emancipator, was correct that somehow this would benefit my health. Otherwise, the only conclusion I could come to was that months of dieting in preparation for the reunion had simply made me daft and demented.

I had to admire Strump, though. Her office brims with medals from thirty-two marathons she has raced, and at fifty-five, the woman radiates health. She took up running at forty-five, a full three years older than me, and became a reflexologist and colonic "emancipator" at fifty. I admired her pluck and dedication, though I questioned some of her other devoutly held beliefs. Could colonics really free the body of toxins, as well as emotional blockages that stymie relationships? While she had sloshed through my intestines, she confessed that her own husband, a physician, thought the whole idea of colonics was nonsense.

"Of course, he's only had 'western' medical training.'" She used her hands to mimic quote marks when she used the word "western." I got her meaning instantly. It's hard to say who has more contempt for whom: holistic healers for the orthodox medical establishment, or the orthodox medical establishment for holistic healers. Antipathy runs deep between the two camps. Perhaps they all need a few high colonics.

"Also, my husband has issues with his father's colon, and so I can never discuss my work with him," Strump said as she gently kneaded my abdomen. I thought about asking what in the world she meant by that, but then thought better of it. Everyone in the holistic healing world felt everyone else had "issues" with something. But a colon? How do you have issues with a colon?

"Please call me anytime if you have any questions or if you feel weak," she told me as I took my empty colon and emptier wallet out of the office. "And remember, eat very lightly today. Fruit and water, perhaps steamed veggies. Try to avoid dairy, meat, wheat, oil, coffee, and the other foods we discussed."

"Um-hmm," I mumbled noncommittally. I was sick and tired of all these people giving me the same laundry list of forbidden foods. And since I had not been allowed to eat for several hours before the procedure, and it was already nearly lunchtime, I silently vowed to head straight for a Starbucks and a chocolate-chip muffin. I had endured enough punishment for one morning.

I'm not at all sure if this will do any good in terms of my weight loss, but I sure don't see the harm in having a clean colon. I'll weigh myself tomorrow and find out.

June 15

I am up a half-pound since yesterday's colonic. Words fail me.

June 18

The kids are completely wired with excitement since school is now out. To celebrate, I took them all for ice cream, and let them choose whatever they wanted. I hadn't been in an ice cream store in a long, long time. I felt strong until the radio began playing, "You Make It Easy" and the store manager had to say "Excuse me, Ma'am!" several times before I realized I was staring catatonically at the tub of Wowie Kazowie Brownie Marshmallow Heaven. My hands were pressed too hard against the glass case, and I saw that my heavy breathing had begun to melt the contents on the other side.

I collected my wits, gave it all over to God, who I still did not believe only created chocolate by accident, and paid for the kids' ice cream. I snapped out of my delirium and didn't order a thing. And it was really okay.

June 22 (eight days before Coop reunion)

Today is my birthday, and my husband and children, the people whom I love more than anyone else in the world, went completely nuts shopping for me. They were very excited when they dragged the large, bulky, heavy bag from the closet to the living room, where I had been invited to sit to receive my bounty. I couldn't imagine what they had hidden in what appeared to be a small suitcase, but when I began to tear open the wrapping paper, it all made sense.

Inside, I found a new canvas gym bag emblazoned with the logo of a major athletic shoe manufacturer. I gushed gratitude to one and all, when one of the boys said, "That's not all there is, Mom. Look inside!"

Oh boy! I thought. Perhaps the gym bag was just a gag, a come-on to something more, shall we say, feminine and luxurious! My heart skipped a beat, and when I dutifully unzipped the bag I did indeed discover a small world of treasures suitable for a gym rat. The kids had all chipped in and bought me a new set of eight-pound weights in purple (my favorite color) and a combination exercise chronograph/heart monitor. The chronograph (with large angled dot matrix display) will tell me how long I exercise, how far I walk or run, and how many calories I burn while doing so. I can also preset the heart monitor to dial 911 if the little machine detects I am in danger of killing myself while getting into shape.

As if all that weren't enough, the kids also bought me a set of six anklet socks, athletic tape for my hands (a real plus on boxing night), a plastic comb, a six-pack of water bottles, and a stick of "powder fresh scent" deodorant. So emotionally stirred by this outpouring, I was incapable of speech.

Jeff smiled devilishly as I extracted gift after gift. This was my payback for all the times I failed to make a decent dinner, take the kids for new shoes, or help type social science reports on the middle ear because I was too busy sculpting my obliques to pay the family any mind.

They had even gone to the vegan bakery and bought an oat-flour carob cake, which served six but weighed twelve pounds. We all took polite bites from the horrendous thing, before giving up and ransacking some frozen cake miraculously leftover from another birthday last March.

After the kids were asleep, Jeff handed me a birthday card with a gift certificate to a fancy store carrying ladies' clothing and lingerie. In his note, Jeff hinted that it was time to retire my oversized Laker's t-shirt I wore as pajamas, perhaps as an athlete might retire a jersey. He held out the hope that I would redeem the certificate as soon as I could fit this task into my busy athletic schedule.

I promised to comply, and went to sleep secure in the knowledge that my family still loved me after all.

June 29

Very little time to write today. Tomorrow is the reunion! Today after the gym I'm going to get my teeth brightened, then off to Lori for a haircut, highlights, and miscellaneous other renovations that become necessary after the age of forty. By the way, my dress arrived a few days ago, and it looks great, as good as it did on my suddenly slenderized virtual model! It's a very simple wraparound dress with a V-neck in a tiny black and white houndstooth print that's on the dressy side of casual. With eight pounds gone, I haven't made my original goal of losing fifteen, but so what? I can do a set of twenty bench presses at fifty pounds! I can do forty sit-ups at a time! I can run a half-mile while singing military cadences and keep my place at the front of the line! I can match Popeye in a spinach-eating contest, though one needs to build up to this slowly. And I can drink almost anyone under the table – provided it's filtered water.

In any event, I hope to deflect whatever attention might go to my still ample hips by having dazzling white teeth, along with a great haircut and make-up. With some luck, I just may still make my goal of being able to see my old pals and be the one to walk away feeling vaguely superior.

June 30

In my wildest dreams, I never would have expected the reunion to be so full of drama, backbiting, intrigue, and bad food. But then again, life is full of surprises. It's already so late at night, but I'm too wired from the party to sleep.

Where do I begin? First, I'll state for the record that in my opinion, I looked absolutely *mah-vah-lous*. Enough old pals from Coop days complimented me on how well I looked to have restored my faith in the public. After I had changed outfits six times and put the finishing touches on my makeup, (a project that had taken a full hour), I stood in front of Jeff, twirled once around, and asked him, "How do I look?" My sport for the evening would be fishing for compliments, and I had just cast the rod for the first time.

"You look fine," he said while not even looking my way. Instead, he was looking in the mirror and performing the only beauty ritual I have ever seen a man perform, namely, slapping on some cologne.

"'*Fine?*' That's all you can say is, '*fine?*'"

Jeff looked at me with a suddenly frightened expression. It had dawned on him that he had just said something wrong, perhaps terribly wrong, without quite knowing what it was. It's tough going for husbands when they realize they have just committed this type of faux pas with their wives. Usually, they have no clue how to extricate themselves.

"I mean, you always look nice when we go out," he said, still looking anxious. "You look really, *really* nice!"

I tried to feel compassion for him. Men can't be expected to understand certain things, and I know he didn't mean any harm.

"You look beautiful! A knockout!" He was reaching for a lifeline, hoping that at any moment, he would grab onto the one that would get him out of deeply troubled waters. "I'll need to keep my eye on you all night, you look so gorgeous!"

"Okay, okay, you can knock it off now," I said. "Let's get going."

But Jeff did not keep his word to keep his eye on me all night. I lost sight of him shortly after we arrived at Bobbi's exquisite home. We couldn't go in right away – first we had to wait in line at the front door to sign the liability waiver she'd had her lawyer prepare. It would have taken us all night to read the forty pages of fine print, so we just dashed off our signatures, indemnifying Bobbi for any accidents or damage to our persons during the party. Right after that, Jeff made a beeline for the bar, where a cache of imported beers and ales sat in tubs of glinting ice. Meanwhile, I quickly spied Lana, whom I hadn't seen in nearly ten years. We hugged and huddled in conversation, while I tried not to let my eye wander in an obvious way as I looked to see if Hartley or Gary had arrived. Both had said they would show.

Lana looked terrific, and when I told her so, she quickly fessed up to having had some recent collagen injections. "You know what they say, Judy," she said with a smile. "After forty, it's all maintenance."

Lana and I exchanged some workout tips, as well as phone, cell and pager numbers, e-mail and snail mail addresses, and made a lunch date for the following week. As we chatted, the doorbell rang, and we watched eagerly to see whom Bobbi would greet next. A couple came in, and I didn't recognize the woman at all. The man looked familiar, but his rounded gut and the obvious lid over what I assumed was a bald pate underneath made him hard to place, until, that is, I saw those mesmerizing blue eyes. It was Gary! The mists of time had been rough on the poor guy!

Soon Lana and her husband, Gary and his wife, and I were all talking chummily, swapping photos of our kids and all agreeing how silly it was for us to have let so many years slide by without getting together. I wondered why Jeff had not reappeared, so I excused myself to go find him. Imagine my shock when I saw him rubbing elbows and imported ale bottles with none other than Jack! I walked over, trying to hide my surprise while accentuating my rouged cheekbones.

"Jack, this is my wife, Judy. Judy, this is Jack. He's a personal trainer at your gym. Maybe you've seen him there," Jeff said. Jack looked at me with a flash of recognition, a flash that was still overwhelmed by uncertainty.

"Sure. You know me, Jack. I'm the one who can do twenty reps of fifty pounds on the bicep machine."

"Of course," Jack's muscles seemed to have been set on "autoflex," since they bulged all by themselves, even when he didn't move. "I didn't recognize you in a dress and all made up," he added.

"Understandable," I said. "But I'd recognize you anywhere, Jack." *Even if, God forbid, I saw you wearing a dress and make-up.*

I then learned what brought Jack to the reunion. It turned out that he had begun as Bobbi's personal trainer and had been promoted to her "significant other!" What a small, small world of fitness it is!

Although Jack and Jeff had really hit it off, trading recommendations about favorite foreign beers, I wanted to pull Jeff away before either of them drank so much that they decided to arm-wrestle. Therefore, I took my husband by the hand, as he clutched a bottle of hearty Finnish ale, and led him to the living room, the main hub of activity. We moseyed from one pocket of people to another, reminiscing a little but mostly talking about our rapid-fire paced lives today. I began to feel very silly about my prolonged anxiety over my appearance for the reunion. I looked around and saw the obvious: After twenty years, we *all* looked older. About half had put on noticeable weight, and only Angela, who wore faddish low-slung jeans and a belly-revealing rhinestone-studded t-shirt, managed to still look only twenty-five. I had never cared for Angela, anyway, since she was one of the only Coop members who would actually write her initials on hard-boiled eggs and other personal snacks in the refrigerator. Talk about miserly!

I felt relaxed, but also hungry. I ate very little during the day, having budgeted most of my points for the reunion. As I would quickly discover, I needn't have bothered. When Bobbi invited us all to go out to the patio for the buffet dinner, an instruction I was eager to follow, I discovered that Ingrid and the caterer had rigged the menu with every possible icky food in the world. Almost nothing on the buffet table was recognizably human food, but at least these unpalatable platters came with subtitles on little cards: "Rice balls with umeboshi plums." "Rice paper spring rolls filled with avocado." "Curried peanut soup." I hate avocado. I hate curry. I won't eat anything called "rice paper" – it sounds like stationary. But the real punishment was inflicted by the main course, which included such gastronomic obscenities as baked beans with pineapple (a dish inspired by Demeter, the goddess of some kind of legume), mint chutney, and okra barley stew. If all this hadn't anchored us to our chairs, dessert would have finished the job. I saw very few people brave enough to impale their forks on the currant-almond nut loaf made with triticale flour (a Frankensteinian concoction that would have needed to be weighed on a truck scale), or dip their spoons in a sickening carob coconut ice cream.

Jeff and I stood in line next to Lana and her husband, Chuck. When Chuck looked at the spread, he threatened to report the meal to Amnesty International.

"You mean we paid forty-five bucks a piece for this?" Chuck asked, shaking his head in amazement.

"'Fraid so," Lana said. "Maybe we can cut out early and go to a restaurant."

But if the food itself hadn't caused me to lose my appetite, Ingrid's welcoming speech would have. It is a speech that will forever live in infamy, and one that proved to me that no good deed ever goes unpunished.

Ingrid stood up in front of the assembled guests and began innocently enough. She thanked everyone for coming, as well as Bobbi for hosting the reunion at her home, Lana for helping print and mail invitations, and me for my help in coordinating the event. She then promised that after dessert, we'd have a chance to each share what we felt our greatest accomplishments had been over the past twenty years. (You can take the woman out of the encounter group, but you can't take the encounter group out of the woman.) That's when my mortification began. Ingrid thought she'd just give one example of this kind of accomplishment, using me as an Exhibit A.

Ingrid, my old friend, fitness inspiration and nemesis, announced in front of everyone, "Most of you probably don't realize this, but ever since I told Judy about this Coop reunion last fall, she has made a dedicated effort to improve her health and fitness, and I for one am proud of her. As someone else who, like Judy, never used to think twice before chugging down diet sodas in the morning and feasting on the type of junk food manufactured by multinational agribusinesses that line their pockets by shortening our lives and throwing our yin and yang into total disequilibrium, I want to salute Judy for setting this great example."

I sat there, stunned and furious. I dug my freshly manicured nails into Jeff's legs as my only alternative to getting up and clawing Ingrid's eyes out in front of everybody. Incredibly, it got worse.

"So, even though I know that despite her hard work, Judy did not manage to completely kick the sugar habit, or the chocolate habit, or lose the fifteen pounds that she had set as her goal by this evening, I am proud of her achievements in personal growth. Judy, even though I consider myself something of an expert in matters of health and wellness, I want you to know that even *you* have inspired me through your efforts. And now, I hope you will all enjoy the macrobiotic meal we have had prepared for you. We'll reconnect again after dessert for what I just know will be a meaningful dialogue!"

If only Hermoine Strump had been there, with her speculum and hose, I would have paid a lot of money to have her use it to emancipate every internal organ in Ingrid's macrobiotic body, right there on the patio. If only I had brought my boxing gloves, I would have demonstrated my new and improved upper right hook and dispatched Ingrid without mercy. While I sat, still frozen in my chair, Jeff patted my knee under the table, an effort to reassure me that the world had not just ended. It was, I knew, also a warning for me not to get up and doing anything rash.

"Don't worry," Jeff said to me. "Everyone here knows she's a nut."

"If I break her legs right now, do you think I could get off on a temporary insanity defense?" I asked. "Eating curried peanut soup has been known to do that to people."

"We can leave if you want."

"No. I'm too mortified to move. I think I'll just sit here and beam hate chakras toward her for the rest of the night."

"I will too."

"Me too," Chuck and Lana both said.

Fortunately, at that very moment, inspiration struck, and I began to taste the revenge I would take on Ingrid. It would not need to be violent to be effective. But it would be delicious. I rose from my chair.

Jeff grabbed my arm and said, "Where are you going?"

"I have to make a phone call. I'll be right back." I knew I sounded calm as I said this, perhaps *too* calm. Jeff looked alarmed. Still, I took my cell phone from my purse and crossed the patio to go into the house. I walked quickly and with purpose. Even Jack, who cast a giant shadow as he stood in the opening where the French doors led from the house to the yard, stepped aside for me. When I returned a few minutes later, Jack stopped me by planting one enormous paw on my shoulder.

"If you want, I'd be happy to offer Ingrid some personalized instruction at the gym. I'll show her the wrong way to use all the machines. It'll serve her right."

"That's very generous of you, Jack. I'll leave it to you to decide, but if you make an appointment with her, let me know. I'll want to watch from across the room."

"Will do. You know, that's just the kind of guy I am."

I returned to the table, feeling better by the minute. In about a half-hour, Ingrid would get her comeuppance.

"Where did you go? What did you do?" Jeff asked, still clearly worried.

"With one simple phone call, I arranged to solve several problems all at once. You'll see soon. Relax. I didn't slash her tires or anything." I began to feel giddy in anticipation.

Chuck, who worked in computer technology, said, "Judy, if you like, I could arrange to send thousands of pieces of spam to Ingrid's computer. Just say the word."

"I'll sign her up for every book-of-the-month club in the country. She won't know what hit her," Lana said. They both seemed buoyed by the notions.

Even Bobbi, who barely knew me, leaned over and whispered that she'd be willing to set up a meeting with Ingrid and give her terrible investment advice. Sally, an alumna who worked in a breast imaging center, chipped in with an offer to arrange a free mammogram for Ingrid, during which she would press the plates down just a little too hard.

I must say, this outpouring of righteous indignation on my behalf touched me to the core. This was what all reunions should be about! Friends proving their friendship and loyalty, across the years and across the miles! I felt truly loved! While the alumni picked sadly at their food, Lana and I just sat drinking our mineral water, while our husbands nursed their beers. We all refused to eat anything. I heard Chuck's stomach growling, and he told Lana he had had enough and wanted to go get some real eats. I begged him to try to hold out for a few more minutes.

Thankfully, very shortly thereafter I heard the bell ring in the house. Bobbi again dutifully flitted inside to answer. She came back out to the patio again quickly, looking puzzled.

"Did anybody here order a bunch of pizzas?" she asked as a young man balancing a large, rectangular insulated red bag stood next to her.

"Of course not!" Ingrid said. "Who would have ordered pizzas at a catered dinner?" I detected a note of panic in her voice.

"I did," I said, standing. "Sixteen pizzas, half with extra cheese. Just lay them down right here," I said, patting my hand on our clear table. "Everybody's welcome to dig in!"

Jeff laughed and gave me a kiss. People began to applaud and hoot and holler. Several alumni immediately dumped their pathetic portions into the garbage and bolted over to our table for some piping hot, white flour crust pizza.

"Brilliant!" Gary said, piling three slices on his plate and giving me ten bucks as a contribution.

If I do say so myself, at that point the party really got going. I collected donations from the grateful Coop alumni for the pizzas (eventually making a small profit), and cast a triumphant, vaguely superior glance at Ingrid, who looked utterly dyspeptic. I put a piece of pizza on a plate and walked over to her.

"Want a piece? It's delicious," I said.

"No thank you," she said frostily.

"Are you sure? It's got extra broccoli."

Ingrid just stared at me. I shrugged, then took a big bite. I chewed slowly, looking her straight in the eye. After I swallowed politely, I said, "Great party, isn't it?" I then shimmered away in my new dress.

Back at our table, Jeff and I were having a wonderful time. Jack and Bobbi joined us, and even Titanic Triceps himself, who had professed dismay when I told him I ate mango for breakfast, filled a plate with four slices – extra cheese. It did my heart good to see a man eat like that.

The doorbell rang again.

"Maybe that's dessert!" Chuck said, and people looked at me expectantly. Only I knew it wasn't. I had timed my dessert delivery not to arrive for another hour. No need to eat so much so fast, after all.

In another moment, Bobbi came out and announced, "Hey everybody, look who's here! It's Hartley and his friend, Robin!"

Hartley! In the past hour, having gone from utter and complete mortification to triumph and success, I had forgotten all about him! Hartley looked as if he forgot to stop the timer on a tanning salon machine. He was dressed expensively, and wore a barely post-pubescent girl on his arm. As he scanned the patio, he naturally gravitated toward the biggest crowd, now huddled around our table with the pizzas. We'd already torn through half the boxes.

Hartley saw me as he approached, with his girlfriend Robin tottering after him uncertainly in spiky heels. I felt my heart race, and rose as he arrived at our table.

"Judy! You look fantastic! You haven't changed a bit!" he said. I just smiled and said, "Hartley, meet my husband, Jeff. Jeff, Hartley."

The two men shook hands, and then Hartley said hello to the rest of the gang. Hartley and Robin sat down at the table next to ours, where I could study him from a safe distance. In profile, it appeared that Hartley had undergone cosmetic surgery – he was not the owner of that aquiline nose back in college. And Lana, who was also trying to get a read on my old flame, whispered to me that she could swear he had had botox injections. She suspected this because when anybody said things that he claimed surprised him, he didn't look surprised – a telltale sign!

I quickly deduced that Hartley's girlfriend Robin was a silly little souvenir he must have picked up sometime after divorce number two. After he dropped out of school, Hartley had remained in New York, trying his hand at acting. And, despite his good looks and a made-up sounding name, his career fizzled out. Although he eventually became a successful talent manager, his personal life was a wreck, his tan was all wrong, he had one kid in rehab, and was dating a girl who was probably still in driver's ed. So, this is what had become of the serial Lothario who had dumped me two decades ago! As my grandmother would have said, "Feh!" I felt grateful that he broke my heart when he did, since if he hadn't done it then, he surely would have done so later, when he traded me in for the baby-sitter. Anyway, I had Jeff, a wonderful husband and father for nearly fifteen years! What was an artificially sleek nose and hair transplants compared to that? What a glorious moment when I saw Hartley sneak several glances in my direction during the evening. Was that wistfulness in his eye, or just a touch of hay fever? I chose to think it was the former. Lana also saw him looking my way repeatedly. We smiled and slapped each other's hands with aggressive "high-fives."

When we were full of pizza, a chastened Ingrid tried to get everyone's attention. She was trying to make good on her threat to make us talk about our accomplishments and sing "Kumbaya." No one paid attention. We were too busy forming plans for an ongoing Coop virtual reunion web site, where we could post alumni updates, photos, and chats. Computer-savvy Chuck offered to head up the site. Ingrid moped off to the side with a single Coop alumnus who had taken pity on her. I saw them commiserating over some leftover okra stew. I guess Ingrid could console herself knowing that the peppers and onions on our pizzas had undoubtedly been sprayed and coated with toxic pesticides.

The evening ground to a natural conclusion, the pizzas having been nibbled down to the last crust. I clinched my status as Most Valuable Player for the reunion when the ice cream arrived, and we all dispatched dessert with much the same speed and vigor as we used to do as undergrads. Jeff and I then departed. After the debacle on the patio, I felt absolutely heady with how well the evening ended. I had stuffed my Palm Pilot with a dozen phone numbers of my newly reacquainted friends. All this friendship got to be a bit much even for me, however, when Jack and Bobbi invited Jeff and me to join them for tennis doubles on the weekend. I demurred, never having played tennis and not wishing to invite any athletic competition with them. But Jeff, who was a bit swacked from the beers, agreed to a few sessions at the gym with Jack.

I guess I should have bought the family membership at The Sculpted Self.

NOVEMBER

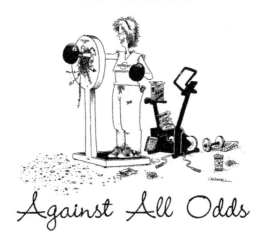

Against All Odds

November 3

Last week a poster in the gym locker room caught my eye. It said, "What are YOU getting in shape for?" The poster displayed photos of four females in fine fettle, each in a Sheriff's Department uniform, packing heat. I wondered what it signified that the state had been reduced to recruiting new police officers in the ladies' locker room of The Sculpted Self – were we that desperate to establish order in the streets? In any event, there it was. The government dangled the enticing opportunity for me (yes, me!) to begin an exciting, rewarding career in law enforcement, joining the ranks of those such as Heidi Brummell, highway patrol officer. Heidi beamed a "She's got to have it" confidence sitting on her motorcycle, taking a breather in between high-speed chases down the Interstate. Or, I could follow in the footsteps of Latisha LaCross, who with one hand on her holster was primed for action. She had the kind of "can-shoot" spirit that I have always liked in a correctional officer.

Steely-eyed Candace Tjorston, hostage negotiator, struck just the right note of style and substance in her flak jacket and coral lipstick. I wonder if Candace takes her daughter to "Take Your Daughter to Work Day" even while she's in the midst of tense negotiations with a suicidal serial rapist. ("I can't get you crayons right now, Cheyenne, Mommy's trying to keep that nice man over there from blowing his brains out.") Finally, there was detective Olivia Crawford, her badge freshly shined, her desk neat. She exuded the kind of saucy satisfaction that can only result from helping throw criminals behind bars, where they would then have to answer to Latisha LaCrosse. While I stood there, combing my hair with the plastic comb the kids had given me for my birthday last summer, I studied these modern-day heroines, each making her own contribution to keeping the streets safe from hooligans. Had they, too, begun these exciting careers by doing sets of twelve leg lunges and roundhouse kicks at a gym?

It occurred to me that as a mother of three sons and one daughter (all of whom had been referred to euphemistically by outsiders as "spirited"), I *already* had considerable on-the-job training required for all of these occupations. After all, how much of a stretch is it really to go from careening down the city streets in a minivan desperate to find the closest available bathroom open to the public for a desperate six-year-old squirming in the back bench and screaming, "I can't WAIT!" to the skills required of a highway patrol officer? And surely, if I could enforce a time-out on a child who had taken a bite out of the neighbor's kid's ankle and had figured out how to break down the door using only a Fisher-Price drill and a pogo stick, patrolling the nightly lock-down in an adult detention center seemed like a piece of cake.

As for the job of hostage negotiator, puh-*leeze*. A day doesn't go by around here without someone getting hammerlocked by a sibling for some supposed crime or other. Just the other day, I successfully negotiated the release of my youngest child, who had violated the "No-Fly Zone" over the computer during a fiercely competitive game of computer chess. She landed up tied and bound after showing one of her brothers a neat way to get the other brother in checkmate, just by moving one rook. The checkmated brother resented this intrusion, resulting in the hostage-taking. After only twenty-five minutes, I secured my daughter's freedom for the small price of a new basketball.

Yes, given my curriculum vitae, I felt eminently qualified to protect and to serve the people of my state. My body, while still loping toward middle age, is now sculpted enough so that I don't think I'd be laughed out of the running. (Besides, under a bulletproof vest, who would ever know that my abs are still a little flabby?) The only catch is that the job entails certain sacrifices, such as moving to another county, and I don't think I'm up for such a long-distance carpooling schedule. While I was attracted to the drama of these jobs, however, I reluctantly decided that I was unlikely to begin sporting a hip holster any time soon. Still, it's always nice to be asked.

November 10

Last night I made a dramatic announcement to my family. I chose the dinner hour to break the news, or, to be more precise, the three-minute span during the dinner hour when everyone is still at the table.

"Guess what, everybody? I'm going to become a personal trainer!"

I stood there, filled with pride, oblivious to the fact that I was still wearing the ankle weights and waist trimmer ("one size fits most") from my afternoon workout. The responses to my announcement were completely underwhelming. Jeff looked puzzled; two of the kids seemed not to have heard; one suddenly yowled in pain because the wire on his braces had just popped out, poking him in the cheek, and the last kid arched an eyebrow cynically while rolling his eyes – a well-worn expression for a young teen.

"You're going to do *what?*" Jeff asked.

"I'm going to become a personal trainer. You know, a certified fitness instructor."

"I knew Mom was becoming certifiable," the teen said, heaping another serving of lasagna on his plate.

"Sarcasm will get you nowhere, which includes the party this weekend for which you need me to chauffeur you both ways," I parried. Parrying is a highly useful sport to master with teens. Keeps the brain alert. "Anyway, *I* think it's a great idea. It came to me yesterday when I went to Cardio Cosmos."

"How did you get in there?" Jeff asked. Cardio Cosmos was L.A.'s most exclusive gym.

"A buddy from The Sculpted Self gave me a guest pass. I always wanted to try it." And who wouldn't? Cardio Cosmos is so ritzy they employ a whole squadron of men in tuxedos to valet park the steady stream of Mercedes-Benzes, Porsches and Hummers that roll in from dawn till nearly midnight every day. The average car in their parking lot costs more than all the cars I have ever owned or will ever own in my entire life. I described how I was forced to keep driving through the valet lane after I saw the shocking prices for this service, not to mention the sneer on the valet's face when he saw my wheels.

"You'd think the guy had never seen a minivan with a compost experiment in the back seat before," I said. "I didn't need an uppity valet." I eventually hid my car several blocks away, near the other undesirable vehicles.

Even the kids perked up when I described this posh pavilion. They were eager to know if I saw any of the Los Angeles Lakers there, as some of them are known to be members. (It's possible, but then again, everybody there looked like a professional athlete to me.) Even though I had been to a lot of gyms in the past year, Cardio Cosmos absolutely blew my sweat socks off. Essentially, it's a Ritz-Carlton with Stairmasters and a thousand weight machines. Their Olympic-sized swimming pool is staffed by Olympic athletes. Their café serves eel sushi. So many celebrities work out there that women go to the salon to get made up — *before* their Hard Rock Kickboxing class begins! It is even bigger than Muscle Mart, and for all I know may have its own municipal government.

I told them about my grueling Ultimate Body workout and spiced it up with a true story. During class, an impeccably made-up woman was humiliated when a hidden piece of foam boinged right out of her halter top during a set of bicep curls. The foam projectile whooshed lightly, landing on a step platform in the row in front of her. (And men wonder why it takes women so long to get dressed!) Red-faced and half-stuffed, the victim of this unexpected foamectomy grabbed her fallen falsie and her keys and hightailed it out of the room, not even bothering to put away her weights or step platform. Still, it's hard for me to muster pity for people who come to these gyms with *fake* padding.

After the class, I saw several dozen personal trainers standing around by the weight machines, exuding the glow of health. They all wore black t-shirts identifying them as "PERSONAL TRAINER," in heavy, urgent-looking block letters. I wandered over to a counter where the gym sold its own patented brand of protein shake mixes (they even deliver to your home with a minimum purchase), as well as private sessions with a trainer. A middle-aged woman standing nearby was studying a wall filled with glamour shots of the entire battalion of trainers, lingering for a long while over one photo of a brawny Adonis.

"I'll take ten sessions with him," the woman told a man working the counter, pointing to the photo with a gleam in her eye.

"He looks. . . *qualified!*" Her voice had a husky timbre.

On the far end of that same counter, I was startled to see a big old glob of lumpy, bumpy rubber in a sickly shade of yellow. Next to it was a sleek, smooth reddish rubber slab. I poked both the slabs.

"What's this?" I asked a peppy young trainer named Ivy. She identified the yellow bumpy slab as a model of five pounds of fat, its red sleek neighbor was a model of five pounds of muscle. I looked at the fat model and thought, Wow! I lost two of these! I mentioned this to Ivy, who then said, "I also lost twenty-five pounds last year and got into shape. When my friends started asking me for help, I decided to become a trainer."

At that moment, I had a brainstorm. Ivy had just given me a smashing idea, far superior than becoming a hostage negotiator for the Sheriff's Department. I grabbed Ivy's arm. "What did you say?"

"I said, I decided to become a personal trainer to help my friends get in shape. And now I work here."

I had often seen flyers at The Sculpted Self recruiting candidates for fitness instructor programs. Only a year ago I would have had a better chance of being hired as a physics professor at MIT than I would have of becoming a personal trainer. But that was before I threw the gauntlet down in front of myself, just barely missing a kneecap, and set out to discover if, somewhere under this chocolate-addicted, overly padded and out-of-shape body, I might unearth something resembling a reasonably fit woman.

This took months and months of hard work, made tougher by having to listen to sniveling, flawless-looking twenty-five-year-old women at the gym complaining that their abs, which were so solid you could have carved a turkey on them, were not nearly as marbleized as their friends' abs, which were so hard I was amazed they were able to pierce the belly button. These odious females had the audacity to kvetch loudly about how much they hated their bottoms, their breasts, their hips, or some other part of their anatomies, which to me looked as if they had been digitized at a special effects studio. Meanwhile, my abs still looked more like a bowl of rising bread dough than they did the fabled six-pack, with grain perhaps being the only common denominator.

Despite these travails, I never gave up. As Winston Churchill, though not exactly a paragon of physical fitness, once said, "Never give in, never give in, never, never, never, never!" And so I found the new me: trimmer, yet still soft around the edges and still a chocolate fiend, but a true fitness aficionado! This time, exercise had been more than just another cheap fling – it had become a committed relationship. It felt great to be on speaking terms with many muscle groups that had lain dormant for decades. It felt great to hold my own through even the toughest aerobics class.

"Maybe I could do the same thing!" I said to Ivy, my new kindred spirit despite her having an unforgivable eighteen percent body fat. "I'd love to finally learn the difference between a trapezius and a trapezoid, or a quadrilateral and a quadricep, and help my friends as well!" Math and exercise had always been my worst subjects. Maybe now, at least, I would excel at one of them. I felt a surging excitement about this idea, though I confessed to Ivy that I doubted whether I was in good enough shape to qualify. Unlike her, I never did lose all the weight I set out to lose. Those last five pounds have insisted on following me everywhere. I've made peace with my ten-pound loss, and lobbed off enough inches so that even my new, smaller-sized clothes have wiggle room. With the reunion behind me, I don't even bother weighing myself that often anymore. As the Major told me last time I saw him, "It's not what you weigh, it's how you look in the MIRROR!" Strangely, the Major only offered this insight *after* forcing Boot Camp weigh-ins on me.

"Don't worry," Ivy said. "*Anybody* can become a fitness instructor! You can even do it through a correspondence program."

I could have taken offense at this, but didn't. From what I had observed so far, the fitness faithful spent more time polishing their physiques than they did their social skills.

"And so," I continued to my disbelieving family, "today I sent away for my course materials, including a textbook and video. I'll be studying diligently and in a few weeks, I will take my test and get my certification!"

"Are *you* going to try to teach at The Sculpted Self?" my daughter asked. The very thought seemed to embarrass her.

"No. I'm not even good enough to do a lot of things that I'd have to do, such as lunge from side to side on a step platform at mach speed, and I could never lead a spinning class." I didn't explain my other reasons for not aspiring to do this, including my own vanity. I was a far cry from the bewitching babes who taught these classes, though I don't think this last requirement is insurmountable. A few weeks ago I clipped an article about "Big Gulp"-sized fitness instructors who are working in gyms around the country and would even give even Weight Watchers scales a run for their batteries. Despite their girth, these gals can still spin the daylights out of other instructors half their body mass index. When they begin making those spandex halter tops with Teflon reinforcements, I'll consider it.

"I really just want to learn more about physiology," I continued. "After all, some people have already asked me for pointers with exercise, and they find me inspiring. ME!"

The children looked doubtful. I made sure to explain to Jeff that in addition to learning the core essentials of teaching fitness, my course places special emphasis on teaching me about tax deductions for personal trainers.

"Are you going to tell Ingrid?" Jeff asked.

"Humph! I have not spoken to that woman since the reunion and see no reason to resume now," I said. I assume Ingrid is in Oregon or someplace like that, trying to corral poor unsuspecting people into her fruitcakey rebirthing workshops.

"How do you know you can pass?" one of my sons asked.

"Don't you have any faith in me? Listen, I've met a lot of 'certified' instructors, and while they may have six-pack abs, I think that upstairs they may be one can short. How hard can it be? It's an open book test, and this company promises a ninety-three percent 'pass' rate. Besides, there's also an essay section, which is the one area where, if I do say so myself, I am sure I will shellack the competition. Grammar counts. No one will ever catch me mistaking a bicep curl for a tricep curl anymore," I said.

With all this studying under my pedometer belt, I told them, I'll become the neighborhood neuromechanics nabob! "I might even clear out the garage and build a little mini-gym in there," I said.

"I'm all for that," Jeff said. "I'm tired of getting whacked in the head by that stupid door gym you installed in our closet. While you're at it, you can move all your other weights, platforms, chin-up bar and other exercise stuff. Maybe I'll have room for my shoes again."

I was glad that Jeff realized how my plan would benefit him directly. And a private place to work out other than my room would be a godsend. More times than I can count, I have been in the middle of doing an exercise video, only to have the kids all march in, demanding that I immediately help them find the square root of 159, or insisting that I help find a box of Popsicles, since everybody except for one kid got one. Sometimes they'd just pick up my weights and wave them around menacingly, or watch me exercise and compare my movements unfavorably with those of the video instructor.

My head was swimming with ideas for names of classes I'd lead in my little private gym: "Empa-Thighs," "Dare to Derriere," "Bareable Arms," "Kickboxing Karaoke" and "From Flab to Abs: An Archeological Dig." These would be kinder, gentler classes, taught by someone who has been there, and, in some ways, will always be stuck there.

I admitted to the family that I also loved the idea of having a title that is capitalized: "Certified Personal Trainer."

"But you do capitalize 'Mom,'" noted one kid.

"Only when you want something, as in, 'Mom, can you take me shopping?' It isn't capitalized when referred to generically, and that has always struck me as wrong, somehow." It's pretentious to call myself a "Writer" with a capital letter, especially when my writing income is so pathetically lower case. However, I am already thinking of ways to parlay both skills into something more lucrative, such as a book based on my non-revolutionary diet plan, "Chew Less, Move More." I'd sell copies in my studio, as well as a full line of snacks and drinks, including chocolate (mini sizes only — I don't want to give the wrong message).

"But won't people know you did this by correspondence course?" one of my savvier kids asked.

"Pardon me, but we prefer to call it 'distance learning.' And no, my certificate will *not* indicate this detail at all. No one needs to know that I never left the house to demonstrate to any live person that I know how to lift a barbell without throwing my entire lower lumbar region into acute shock. So I'll thank everyone to keep this information in this room."

"Hey, maybe if you get good enough, you can work for Jack," Jeff teased. Jeff had trained a few times with Jack, but with four kids to clothe and feed, our income could not support both of us becoming gym rats.

I hardly think I'll ever end up on Jack's payroll. After all, this scheme of mine is already implausible enough. Who ever would have thought that a weight-lifting washout like me would feel antsy if three days went by without exercising?

Yes, I saw terrific potential in my idea of building my own little fitness empire at home. Not that I would ever give up going to The Sculpted Self completely. I love my Latin Dance and Extreme Cardio-Kickboxing classes – the music, the energy in the room, and even those adorable, strong women who inspire me with their strength. And sometimes, it just feels good to work those clanging machines for my hips and arms, which I know are destined to always be pudgy. Strong, but pudgy.

By the end of the evening, Jeff and the kids had become used to another one of my fanciful notions, and I celebrated the launch of my new venture with a two-point chocolate "Skinny Cow" ice cream bar.

Tomorrow I may begin an outline of my breakout bestseller, *Chew Less, Move More*. Look, crazier things have happened.

Carpool Tunnel Syndrome:
Motherhood as Shuttle Diplomacy

From Bil Keane, creator of *The Family Circus:*
"While my cartoons are a quick-take on typical family life, Judy
Gruen picks up where I left off. I thank the good Lord she's not
drawing a newspaper comic. Get into this carpool.
You'll enjoy the ride."

From Chris Erskine, columnist, *Los Angeles Times*
"*Carpool Tunnel Syndrome* will make you laugh with recognition. Judy
Gruen has the same wacky touch as Erma Bombeck."

Parenting advice overload got you down? Relax! Judy Gruen is a
parenting guru unlike any other! In this nearly fact-free book,
Gruen suggests wacky but wise parenting tricks based on her
in-the-trenches experience as a mother of four kids and two hamsters.
She'll teach you how to hide successfully from the PTA, how much
to pay the National Guard to baby-sit, and when a triple hot fudge
sundae is required for mental health.

Recommended for any mom who
thinks of herself as dressed up because she
yanked the Mickey Mouse glow-in-the-dark
bandage off her finger and ran a diaper wipe
behind the earlobes, *Carpool Tunnel Syndrome*
has got moms (and dads!) laughing about
overzealous parents at Little League games,
cheap imported toys that start beeping at 2:00
a.m., and bizarre pediatric ailments that make
children too sick to go to school, including
"itchy right eyebrow" and "fat hair."

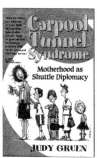

ISBN 1-891400-31-2
Retail Price $13.95
Published by Champion Press, Ltd.

Off My Noodle

Humorist Judy Gruen now offers a free antidote to mirthless Mondays
with her new semi-monthly email humor column, *Off My Noodle*. To
subscribe or learn more log on to www.judygruen.com

About the Author

Judy Gruen's first book, *Carpool Tunnel Syndrome: Mother hood as Shuttle Diplomacy*, catapulted her from com plete literary obscurity to only partial literary obscurity. A resident of Los Angeles, Gruen continues to go to the gym, despite the close proximity of too many women with annoyingly toned arms. She will still follow you anywhere if you promise her a Hershey bar. Her humor has been published in *Woman's Day*, *Ladies Home Journal*, and the anthologies *101 Damnations: The Humorists' Guide to Personal Hells* (St. Martins) and *More Mirth of a Nation* (HarperCollins).

Visit Judy's web site at www.judygruen.com